M. Dombrowsky

X-Ray X-pertise —
from A to X

X-Ray X-pertise —
from A to X

Ray Sherman, D.C.
Felix Bauer, D.C.

Published by

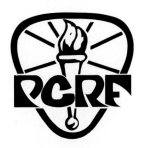

Parker Chiropractic Research Foundation
Box 40444
Fort Worth, Texas 76140

PREFACE

We were so struck by the quality of radiographs and the wide-ranging completeness of *X-Ray X-pertise — from A to X* that we accepted the manuscript as the first book, outside of our own publications, ever to be printed by the Parker Chiropractic Research Foundation printing department. Too, when I asked Dr. Russell Erhardt his advice on our printing this book, he said, "Anything Drs. Ray Sherman and Felix Bauer create on x-ray couldn't help but be worth printing, buying and studying; they are among the best." Those who understand what it takes to read, correct, edit, typeset, proofread, design, print and bind a book of this nature can triple that estimated effort for this technical-made-simple *X-Ray X-pertise —from A to X*, and then be about half aware of what has gone into this mammoth project for a period of two years.

But we would do it again, for I am very much interested in the continuous upgrading of chiropractic radiographic skills and knowledge, and feel certain *X-Ray X-pertise — from A to X* will make a major contribution, not only to all student and practicing chiropractors the world over, but for the thousands yet to come — worldwide.

Here are reasons why PCRF printed this book, and why my name is here as author of its preface.

The book is written for the practitioner and the clinician, not for the academician or theoretician.

Its useful information ranges from basic explanations for the student x-ray user to how-to checks for the seasoned operator.

This book provides material that is useful to an x-ray user in any stage of radiographic progress.

It is written to be easily read and understood.

A chiropractic student could read this one book and have good grounding in radiology. He/she would have the knowledge to take good radiographic films while issuing minimal radiation dosages.

There are many examples of problem-solving (in **Practical Perspectives**) whereby an x-ray user can check the functioning of his equipment . . . perhaps saving a $100-$200 service call several times a year.

The book is a great guide for a new practitioner just setting up his x-ray department.

The book is excellent for chiropractors to give to radiologists, radiographic technicians, etc. It is "state of the art" spinal imaging, and it shows other professionals our responsible position in regard to x-ray.

From my experience, it is unfortunately true that too many inferior x-rays are taken. There is no longer any excuse for this; *X-Ray X-pertise — from A to X* tells operators how to take quality radiographs with reduced radiation, without spending an excess amount of time.

As our colleagues take superior radiographs, government, insurance and other involved instrumentalities will have improved relations with our profession. This diligent x-ray improvement effort by our Australian cousins, I'm told, has in their country improved this situation. The government there now knows that the chiropractors are not amateurs; that they are serious as a group and responsible about quality spinographic work.

With this book, there's little question that the DC can be more confident in his office and in his community. If he is doing quality x-ray work, he is pleased to refer, when needed, more patient's films to other professionals when the patient has, for example, pelvic metastases . . . he no longer has to parrot—at least for professional reasons—"The films remain the property of this office," etc. As well, the professional people in the community give you the respect deserved for quality work, often by increased referrals. One is more a Doctor of Chiropractic in people's eyes. Following the advice contained in this book, certainly will bring about an elevated professional image, to say nothing of improved interpretation skills. The man who takes better quality films and knows he is issuing less radiation ultimately will take more x-rays. Inexorably his income will increase . . . from reading and applying skills learned from X-Ray X-pertise — from A to X although this is not, of course, in and of itself an acceptable yardstick for consideration.

Better quality films yield an increased level of service rendered to patients. Simply, this can mean — among many other benefits — fewer malpractice possibilities . . . from reading X-Ray X-pertise — from A to X.

The BCB (Bilateral Compression Band), the DEF (Density Equalizing Filtration), the gonadal shields, the cervical head steadiers, all are refinements in radiographic procedures.

Using the nomogram printed in this modern book — and following the simple instructions — allows every DC and also the clinical CA to calculate easily the radiation exposure received by the patient from any and all spinal x-ray examinations. It doesn't matter if the patient is a janitor or a physicist — the informed reader of X-Ray X-pertise — from A to X can discuss radiation with confidence.

Ever since "Three Mile Island," there has been an awareness of radiation in the public's mind. If we are "doing the right thing" and know we are, we can refute any and all criticism of chiropractic spinography. Knowledge and facts are power. We can talk with confidence about radiation in our practices and in our communities . . . with the knowledge gained in X-Ray X-pertise — from A to X.

I hope each of my colleagues will say, "I'm buying this book because I'm prideful enough to want to take quality radiographs — for professional, personal and even egoistic reasons. For I'd rather pattern my radiographs after the best rather than the mediocre. Like my chiropractic care, my x-ray films are the best."

Here are a number of questions I found X-Ray X-pertise — from A to X answered:

What is the best grid for spinal imaging requirements?

Should you shoot from 100cm (40") or 200cm (80")?

What should the capacity of your x-ray generator be?

How often should intensifying screens be replaced?

Are graded screens worthwhile?

High or low kilovoltage: which is best?

How safe is your safelight?

How can you avoid expensive x-ray tube replacement?

Which techniques issue the least amount of radiation?

Do you need a fluorescent light in your darkroom?

Who determines which equipment you will purchase — the x-ray distributor or you?

What is the easiest way to test for bucky shudder?

Will quantum mottle spoil your films?

Where do 90% of radiographic errors occur?

Which is for you — automatic or manual processing?

What is the simplest way to calculate the amount of radiation issued for each and every exposure?

Are you proud of your films when they are sent out for interpretation or patient referral?

And finally, to those of you who have been my students and learned the principles of Success Consciousness, let me remind you of one of our cardinal rules: "To succeed, you must more than fill your present place. And to more than fill up your present place you must do each day, all you can do that day, doing each separate thing in as nearly a 100% efficient manner as possible in order to impress the subconscious mind with successful experiences. Repeated successful experiences thus follow as a habit of life."

Taking good, clear, easily interpreted x-rays, thus providing quality service to the sick in this area, is decidedly included in this principle.

In closing, let me make one more observation: everything has not yet been learned, said or written about x-rays. That's why I renamed this book *X-Ray X-pertise — from A to X*. Because, as is the phenomenon of God's Universe — there is always more. And we're still searching and researching for the "Y and Z."

—James W. Parker, D.C.

ACKNOWLEDGEMENTS

The authors especially would like to recognize a number of people and concerns without whom this book might never have been brought to fruition. First of all, our thanks go to our wives and families who retired early many nights leaving us to toil over complex things to make them simple; their patience and encouragement was, like always, gracious and understanding. To our hundreds of patients for whom we took thousands of x-rays in search of the causes of their health problems, we are thankful for their patience in often time-consuming specifics in both taking and interpreting their films.

Financial contributions toward manuscript preparation were received from the Canadian Council of Chiropractic Roentgenology, the Ontario Chiropractic Association, the Michigan Chiropractic Council, Weldon Green, Q.C., and C.M.C.C. Class of 1982. This support has been most helpful.

Individuals contributing welcome asistance in our endeavors included Dr. Ron Duncan, Dr. A. Kleynhann, Messrs. J. Churchill, G. Marrin, K. Jackson and A. Smith.

And we must not forget the writer of the preface of this book, Mr. Chiropractor, the one who has pioneered innovations in our profession for nearly four decades, more than almost anyone in this generation, Dr. James W. Parker.

It is he who renamed it X-Ray X-pertise — from A to X and, as expected, based on his history, that title more perfectly encompasses the book's completeness, in that it is almost all here; just the "Y and Z" are still being worked on. And Dr. Parker's ingenious suggestions in reviewing its overall arrangement and accepting it as the first outside project for the Parker Chiropractic Research Foundation's printing department are gratefully acknowledged. Not enough good things can be said of the staff of Parker Foundation for the tireless efforts in proofing, altering and improving the manuscript chapter by chapter, until its final completion. Our special thanks to PCRF's William D. Brown, Ph.D., Director of Education; John Harrah, B.A., Director of Public Relations, PCRF; Kim Hood, overall project coordinator and art director; and to Shirley Eppler, Carol Ann Kerns, Walter Winsett and Sandra Wright for manuscript preparation.

Finally, special thanks should go to Woody Sherman, wife of Dr. Ray Sherman, for her countless hours of assistance, advice, typing and general all-round organizational capabilities.

Felix Bauer, D.C.

Ray Sherman, D.C.

TABLE OF CONTENTS

FOREWORD

For more than twenty years Felix Bauer, D.C., has been endeavoring to improve the quality of spinal radiography and to lessen the amount of radiation issued to the patient during spinal imaging examinations. Dr. Bauer has spent many hundreds of hours engaged in private research in this field. His working methods closely resemble those of Thomas Edison, as he, too, is a practical innovator par excellence. An idea germinates; lengthy thought is followed by practical procedures to develop and test the hypothesis, and then improvements are adopted. Dr. Bauer has tested countless varieties of films, grids, intensifying screens, cassettes, bucky mechanisms, generating apparatus, tube stands, patient immobilizing devices, gonadal shields, filter systems and exposure techniques. All this has been directed toward the twin goals of radiation reduction and heightened final film quality. Neither has he been parsimonious with his knowledge: Over the past twelve years Dr. Bauer has presented his findings freely at seminars and conferences in Australia, New Zealand, Europe and Canada.

The advances made by Dr. Bauer have resulted in a saving of many thousands of Roentgens to thousands of patients of x-ray users. And it is assured that this book will not only assist in bringing about additional reductions in dosages of radiation issued by x-ray users worldwide, but will improve any operation and interpretation of x-rays. The natural consequence of learning the results of Dr. Bauer's tireless research as revealed in X-Ray X-pertise — from A to X is to better serve the sick by superior chiropractic services.

In reading this book you will notice that Imperial and Metric measurements are used interchangeably, units of each system appearing first at various times. It is recognized that the universal employment of metrics is simply a matter of time. Nevertheless, a transitional period exists and we have used terminology for its presumed familiarity. While this usage must be arbitrary to some degree, we hope that its selection enhances assimilation of material presented.

Also, it was decided early on, that except where American and Australian usage and spelling are radically different, the Australian version would be given the nod to preserve the original flavor of the manuscript.

Ray A. Sherman
Sydney, Australia

Chapter **1**

An Introduction to X-Ray

It is right, therefore, that all of those engaged in exposing members of the public to radiation should understand the extent of the hazards and how to reduce them to a minimum in the course of their work.

K. C. Clark, *Positioning in Radiography,* p. 776, 9th Edition, Volume 2, Published for Ilford By William Heinemann, 1973.

In the late 1800's numerous scientists were experimenting with *cathode ray* tubes. Undoubtedly several of these men generated x-rays, as this new form of radiation came to be called, during the study of cathode ray movement within a glass walled tube. In spite of considerable activity in this field none of these individuals realized "x-rays" existed and so ionizing radiation remained unperceived until November 8, 1895. On this day Professor William Konrad Roentgen, then Professor of Physics of the Royal University of Wurzburg, Germany, discovered x-rays. Roentgen noticed that a cardboard screen, covered with a fluorescent material, gave off a faint green light while the Crookes tube was operative. The room had been darkened and the tube was covered with black cardboard so that any unusual occurrence would be visible. Once the initial observation took place it was but a short time before Roentgen realized that the glass wall of the Crookes tube was generating x-rays as it was being struck by electrons.

Professor Roentgen soon discovered that these invisible x-rays were able to penetrate solid objects. Placed between the tube and the fluorescent screen, a 1,000-page text offered no real hindrance to the passage of the new rays. When he introduced his hand into the path of the rays the luminous outline revealed an accurate representation of the bones of his hand. (Figure 1-1)

It seems certain that if Professor Roentgen had not discovered x-rays when he did, it would have been only a brief time indeed before another investigator happened across this exciting new phenomenon. This is not to take anything away from Roentgen, for he was a meticulous worker who made exacting experiments resulting in accurate, reliable observations. By the end of that same year —1895 — Roentgen made known his findings in a paper designated, "UBER EINE

NEUE ART VON STRAHLEN" ("About a New Kind of Ray"). Roentgen is described by Jacob Bronowski as a "kindly father figure." He became "the hero who won the first Nobel prize in 1901."

Within a few days of Roentgen's announcement, Dr. E. H. Grubbé began experimenting with x-rays. Grubbé's activities were such that he developed severe dermatitis in one hand by January, 1896. Several years later the progression of cancer foreordained the amputation of Grubbé's hand. By this time, of course, there were hundreds of reports discussing the harmful effects of ionizing radiation. Ever since the initial investigations and applications of x-ray, its blessings have been mixed: undeniable diagnostic and therapeutic benefits balanced against yet-to-be fully determined somatic and genetic consequences. We will return to radiation, its effects and its reduction in the final chapter.

In the meantime, we trust you will remain fully cognizant of radiation control measures as they appear in the text. In the final analysis lessened radiation dosages are the *raison d'etre* for this book. (Fig. 1-1: Hand, Roentgen.)

The Electromagnetic Spectrum

X-rays are a part of the electromagnetic spectrum which includes infrared and ultraviolet rays, radio waves and visible light rays. X-rays generally conform to the laws governing light but they also have additional properties; e.g., an ability to penetrate matter and to bring about varying degrees of alteration of living tissue. Gamma rays are little different from x-rays, the point of origin being significant. X-rays originate from outside the nucleus while gamma rays commence from within the atomic nucleus.

Electromagnetic radiation has a dual behavior pattern. It travels in undulations much the same as ocean surface waters travel in waves. There is a corresponding *wavelength* for each type of electromagnetic radiation and, of course, a resultant frequency. The undulating wavelengths of x-radiation are approximately one billionth of an inch in length while those of certain radio waves are five miles long. Fig. 1-2 illustrates various electromagnetic radiations and their location within the electromagnetic spectrum.

We have seen how x-ray behaves as a wave. However, this description is not complete. X-ray can respond as a *particle* and these "particles" are called *photons*. We can say that an x-ray exposure consists of bundles or packets of radiant energy, termed photons or quanta (singular quantum). Photons do not always react evenly while being dispersed over the surface of a radiographic film and this bothersome phenomenon leads to what is termed *quantum mottle*.

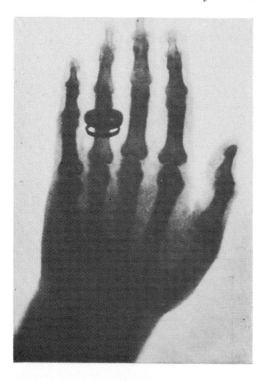

Fig. 1-1 An early radiograph taken by Professor Roentgen on 23 January, 1896.

Production of X-rays

The filament of an x-ray machine is

THE ELECTROMAGNETIC SPECTRUM

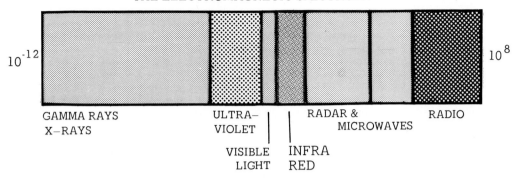

10^{-12} 10^{8}

GAMMA RAYS   ULTRA–   RADAR &   RADIO
X–RAYS   VIOLET   MICROWAVES

VISIBLE   INFRA
LIGHT   RED

Fig. 1-2 — Electromagnetic rays have no mass or electric charge. Fundamentally, they are a form of energy traveling at the speed of light. Their effects result from energy released at the point of interaction with matter.

heated by sending electrical energy through the filament circuit. As the filament temperature increases electrons begin to "boil-off" by what is called *Thermionic emission* and a *space charge* forms near the filament. The space charge is a small cloud of electrons which moves from the cathode to the anode when the exposure button is activated. The electrons must now be stopped promptly, a task accomplished by the anode. At this point electron energy becomes either heat energy or x-ray energy; the former predominates and is responsible for the great lengths that must be taken to properly cool an x-ray tube. Over 99 percent of converted electrons become heat and the diminutive remaining portion becomes ionizing radiation by one of two processes.

Radiation: Bremsstrahlung and Characteristic

Briefly, the loss of electron activity at the anode results in the formation of x-rays labeled either Bremsstrahlung or characteristic radiation. Bremsstrahlung is translated from the German language and means, "braking radiation." As a negatively charged electron passes near a positively charged nucleus the deflection attraction causes the production of an x-ray photon. The second and less common constituent, characteristic radiation, occurs when electrons reach the tube target and dislodge electrons from the inner orbits of atoms in the anode. This causes ionization of the atom and as the atom reverts back to its normal state it releases a photon of x-radiation. There is no characteristic radiation produced beneath 70 kVp. At 80 kVp the characteristic radiation component is ten percent of the total and at 150 kVp it comprises 28 percent of the radiation stream. From this point upwards in the kVp range characteristic radiation gradually disappears.

To repeat, x-rays generated within the diagnostic range are produced via characteristic radiation or via Bremsstrahlung radiation. There are varying energies of x-rays and the lowest energy emitted from the tube is determined by the filtration present. The greatest energy is determined by the kVp utilized.

Current

The current used to power an x-ray generator varies in different parts of the world. In the United States and Canada power is supplied at 120 or 240 volts, 60 cycles per second. In Australia and New Zealand electrical power is supplied at 240 or 415 volts, 50 cycles per second. High voltages are essential to generate x-rays, necessitating transformers to accomplish this task; transformers function on alternating current, explaining why direct current is not used.

Let us return to the matter of cycles per second in alternating current. In the familiar 60 cycle per second power system one complete cycle takes place in 1/60 second, as illustrated in Fig. 1-3. Because a single pulse occupies 1/120 second, exposures must be constructed from multiples of this number allowing for brief exposures of 1/20 or 1/30 second, to the minimum of 1/120 second. Rectification yields 120 cycles per second, allowing the accuracy of an x-ray timer to be checked easily with the aid of a *spinning top*. Of practical importance is the maintenance of an adequate and stable mains supply. The voltage may differ during various periods of the day as related to industrial or domestic requirements. Both the high tension and filament circuits require an intact electrical supply. Radiographic results will be unsatisfactory if the mains current is not up to standard.

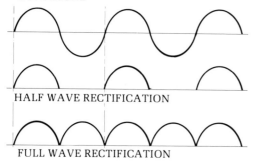

ALTERNATING CURRENT WAVE FORMS
1/60 SECOND

HALF WAVE RECTIFICATION

FULL WAVE RECTIFICATION

Fig. 1-3 Full rectification of the alternating current wave form produces relatively efficient use of electricity in single-phase x-ray generators.

Rectification

Rectification is the method which converts the undulating, wave-like alternating current into direct current. Fig. 1-3 illustrates various forms of rectification. *Half-wave* rectification is inefficient and passe, no longer of interest except as an historical footnote. *Full-wave* rectification is almost universal in application in modern radiography. Certainly, full rectification is necessary for satisfactory spinal imaging requirements. The most common diagnostic generator employed today is the single-phase, fully rectified model.

Rising in popularity is the three-phase generator which produces a more even output than the single-phase generator, as can be readily appreciated from the illustration in Fig. 3-1. We will expand upon pertinent aspects of rectification in Chapter III.

Milliamperage [mA]

Stated simply, *milliamperage* is the current which occurs within an x-ray tube. It refers to the number of electrons which flow during a time period of one second. A well-worn bromide declares that "milliamperage is the quantity of radiation while kilovoltage is the quality of radiation."

The *filament circuit* in an x-ray tube is responsible for propagation of milliamperage. Electrical current reaches the filament, a coiled tungsten wire, and causes it to become heated. When the filament is heated to a sufficient degree, electrons "boil off" by a process known as *thermionic emission*. The resulting space charge passes to the focal spot when the machine's exposure button is activated.

As filament temperature is increased the number of electrons produced increases. In other words, increasing mA increases tube current. An mA of 100 results in an exposure with twice the electrons as an exposure at 50 mA. Since a greater number of electrons traveling to the film means more silver bromide crystals exposed to x-ray photons, the density of a film is controlled by the milliamperage.

The *Reciprocity Law* provides a direct relationship between mA selected and time of exposure in seconds, the product being mAs. Briefly, an exposure of 100 mA for one second will yield 100 mAs; 50

mA for 2 seconds also yields 100 mAs, as does 500 mA for 1/5 second. The Reciprocity Law holds true for screen film exposures between .05 and 5 seconds, the usual time frame for most diagnostic roentgenology.

Because increasing milliamperage produces increased numbers of x-ray photons, a higher mAs technique will produce a greater patient exposure than a higher kVp technique. It is advisable to bear this in mind when establishing technique charts for a particular radiographic unit: reducing patient radiation dosages whenever and wherever possible is always good radiography.

Kilovoltage (kVp)

In an electrical sense voltage is the potential difference existing within a circuit and, of course, kilovoltage is that same difference expressed as thousands of volts. For example, an x-ray generator with a capacity of 125 kilovolts has a capacity of 125,000 volts. (It is understood that international nomenclature now refers directly to kilovoltage, kV, instead of kilovoltage peak, kVp; however, the designation kVp has been in general usage for so long that we will continue this practice.) Originally, kilovoltage peak was not used as a descriptive term; instead the average kilovoltage during a single cycle was measured. There is something to be said for this method because it provides for an easier comparison between x-ray generators. For example, two machines may be quoted as 100 kVp capacity while under the old system one may be 72 kV and the other 66 kV.

Increasing kVp increases the "pressure" within the high tension circuit, thus increasing the energy of the x-ray beam. Higher frequency, shorter wavelength rays are now produced, possessing greater penetration power. Such an x-ray beam allows for a more even penetration of tissue, thus lessening subject and radiographic contrast. Higher kVp produces a

relatively "harder" x-ray beam while low kVp is responsible for what is commonly called a "softer" beam. Increased scatter radiation occurs with higher kVp but, on the other hand, exposure latitude increases at higher kVp levels. (It seems that everything is a "trade-off" in radiography. That is why the quest for diagnostic excellence and lessened patient radiation remains an enduring struggle.)

Some x-ray users prefer low kilovoltage techniques because it is easier to obtain high contrast films at lower kVp settings. The low kilovoltage technique necessitates increased amounts of mAs and, as mentioned earlier, this leads to greater radiation exposure for the patient. Remember that low kVp exposures produce less scatter; therefore, there will be more x-ray energy absorption in the tissues being exposed. Further, high mAs — low kVp techniques create stresses upon

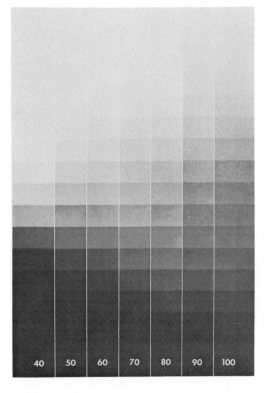

Fig. 1-4 Comparison of contrast at various kilovoltage settings. (Photo courtesy Eastman Kodak Company)

THE INVERSE SQUARE LAW

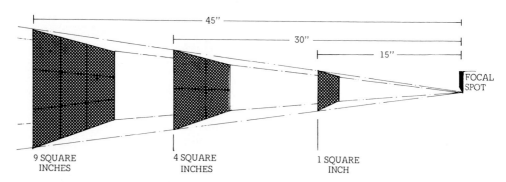

Fig. 1-5 A source of light illuminating 1 sq. in. at a distance of 15″ will illumine 4 sq. in. at 30″ and 9 sq. in. at a distance of 45″. At 30″ the intensity of the light will be 1/4 the intensity at 15″; at 45″ the intensity will be 1/9 the intensity at 15″.

an x-ray tube due to increased heat production at the anode.

Before completing this brief review of kilovoltage the subject of contrast must be summarized. Radiographic contrast comprises subject contrast and film contrast plus the effect of fog resulting from scatter radiation. Kilovoltage affects both subject contrast and scatter production.

High kilovoltage increases the penetration power of photons — as well as increasing the overall number of photons generated — so that there is relatively less differential expressed between various density tissues. Low kilovoltage results in fewer photons reaching the film because they fail to attain complete patient penetration, thus inducing fewer silver sensitization reactions in the development process. High kVp yields low subject contrast, which is labeled *long-scale contrast*, while low kVp yields high subject contrast, labeled *short-scale contrast*. Short-scale contrast progresses rapidly from black to white with few intervening grey steps while long-scale contrast has numerous distinct grey shadings over equal density structures, as illustrated in Fig. 1-4.

The Inverse Square Law

Comprehension of the Inverse Square Law (ISL) is one of the most important

aspects of radiographic knowledge any x-ray user can possess. In fact, without a working familiarity with the simple but often misunderstood ISL, it is quite impossible to become proficient in overall radiation reduction measures.

The Inverse Square Law states that the intensity of x-rays or light is inversely proportional to the square of the distance from the source of the light (Fig. 1-5). Thus, if the focus-film distance (FFD) is increased by a factor of two (doubled) the intensity of a corresponding light is reduced by four (quartered). If the FFD is tripled the intensity of the resulting beam will be reduced to 1/9th of its original intensity. In practical terms this means that an exposure made at 50cm FFD requiring 100 mAs would, from an FFD of 100cm, require an exposure of 400 mAs to maintain the same film density. Likewise, increasing the FFD from 50cm to 150cm would necessitate increasing the exposure from 100 mAs to 900 mAs.

Now this seems to be an inordinately large increase in exposure values. Nevertheless, extending the FFD always results in a decrease of radiation to the patient, other considerations being equal.

The easiest way to depict the practical effects of an increased FFD as it relates to the ISL and patient radiation is with the aid of an illustration, Fig. 1-6. Note diagram (A). The FFD is 20″ (50cm), the patient is 10″ (25cm) thick and so the FSD is 10″ (25cm). In diagram (B) the FFD has been doubled to 40″ (100cm), the patient remains 10″ (25cm) thick and so the new FSD of 30″ (75cm) is three times the original FSD.

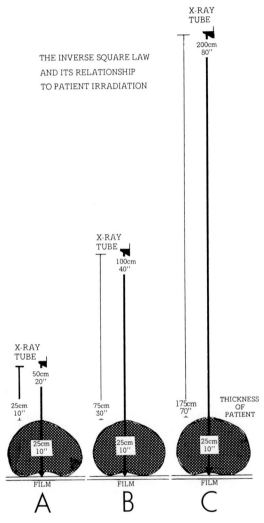

THE INVERSE SQUARE LAW
AND ITS RELATIONSHIP
TO PATIENT IRRADIATION

Fig. 1-6 When the focal spot is moved further away from the patient the FSD increases in relation to the FFD. As explained fully in the text. The result is that patients receive less radiation from longer FFD techniques.

At this point some simple calculations will reveal exactly how a reduction of patient radiation dose occurs. The FFD has doubled from (A) to (B) but the FSD

has tripled. The new FFD requires an mAs value four times that of the first exposure. However, because the FSD has tripled the skin of the patient would have to receive nine times the radiation of the first exposure to maintain its original density.

The same thing stated slightly differently shows that focal-spot-to-film distance has increased 2x while focal-spot-to-patient distance has increased 3x. Maintaining correct density, the radiation exposure to the patient has not increased 9x but only 4x; therefore, the patient only receives 4/9ths the radiation at 40″ (100 cm) as at 20″ (50cm).

Let's proceed one step further: Increasing the FFD to 80″ (200cm) as shown in (C) increases the FFD to 4x that of diagram (A) while the FSD is increased by 7x. According to the rule of the ISL the mAs exposure must be increased 16x for a fourfold increase in focal-spot-to-film distance. The patient, now at sevenfold distance from the focal spot, would need to receive 49x more exposure to be consistent with the ISL. In actual fact the patient does not receive 49x the original exposure in (A) but 16x more exposure. Thus, at an FFD of 80″ (200cm) the patient receives 16/49ths the amount of radiation received at an FFD of 20″ (50cm).

The advantages of long focus-film distances may be evidenced through the application of a simple formula comparing the patient exposure and the film exposure:

Recall that in diagram (A) the FFD was 20″ while the FSD was 10″. The inverse square ratio is:

$$\frac{(\text{Focus-Film Distance})^2}{(\text{Focus-Skin Distance})^2} = \frac{(20)^2}{(10)^2} = \frac{400}{100} = 4.0$$

In diagram (B) the FFD was 40″ and the FSD was 30″. The inverse square ratio is:

$$\frac{(\text{FFD})^2}{(\text{FSD})^2} = \frac{(40)^2}{(30)^2} = \frac{1600}{900} = 1.77$$

In diagram (C) the FFD was 80″ and the FSD was 70″. The inverse square ratio is:

$$\frac{(FFD)^2}{(FSD)^2} = \frac{(80)^2}{(70)^2} = \frac{6400}{4900} = 1.30$$

The illustrations in Fig. 1-6 are elementary for ease in explanation; there are other factors to consider in actual radiographic situations. No allowance has been made for the space between the patient and the film. With an upright bucky it is often possible to place the patient within one or two centimeters of the film. In tabletop applications the bucky apparatus sometimes causes the film to be four, five or more centimeters beneath the patient. This causes magnification and unsharpness as well as bringing the patient closer to the x-ray tube. Positioning the patient closer to the tube insures that a higher skin dose enriches that individual.

Astute readers may observe that increasing the FFD also increases the area of skin that is irradiated on the tube side during an exposure. It is true that the skin entrance field is smaller than a short FFD, but the increased skin entrance field of a long FFD is commensurate with an increased amount of available patient information. There is less magnification of bodily structures in a long FFD technique, thus more of the osseous skeleton will be included within the field of view. Two additional benefits of tele-radiography are improved film detail and reduction of body-part distortion.

The evidence is incontrovertible: increasing the distance between the tube and the film — and the patient, of course — reduces the radiation dose to the individual being examined.

It is our conviction that films, especially lumbosacropelvic views which include or are in proximity to the gonads, should not be taken from the usual distance of 40″ (100cm). Instead, they should be taken from a minimum of 60″ (150cm) or 72″ (182cm) but preferably from 80″ (203cm). Eighty inch techniques should become standard and the conventional, prevailing techniques of filming from "forty inches" should be discontinued wherever possible. The benefit to patients from this one step would be conspicuous in data relevant to exposures received by various population groups.

The horizontally disposed bucky table has the operational disadvantage of a restricted FFD: the height of most tube columns precludes utilization of distances beyond 48″ (120cm). Other than this fact, and a generous dollop of professional inertia, there seems little reason for persevering with the 40″ FFD.

Modern x-ray generators and tubes should be of a standard able to cope with the demands of 200 cm FFDs without breaking down or expiring earlier than anticipated. In the early days of diagnostic roentgenology short focus-film distances were necessary because of equipment inadequacies. It simply was not possible to extend FFDs to 200 cm with the equipment that was available in most facilities. Now that competent generators and larger tubes are available — and have been for several years — it seems that progress in the radiographic world has not kept pace with developments in radiographic equipment.

Half-Value Layer

The half-value layer (HVL), or half-value thickness as it often is referred to in Europe, is the amount of attenuation of a particular material which reduces the intensity of a given x-ray beam by 50 per cent. HVLs are used to describe the quality of an x-ray beam and governments are moving toward the adoption of HVL standards in regulating beam quality. Within the kVp ranges used for conventional diagnostic radiology the beam attenuator is almost always a millimetric thickness of aluminum. For example, at 100 kVp an HVL of 2.7 might be considered acceptable whereas an HVL of 2.2 would be unacceptable. The fact that only

2.2mms of aluminum is necessary to cut the beam's strength by 50 per cent indicates that the stated x-ray tube's potential is inadequate. Half-value layers do provide a concept of the penetrating ability of an x-ray beam.

A beam that has been reduced to its first HVL is "harder" than before it was filtered. In like manner so is a beam further hardened as it is reduced to its second HVL. It is not that more high-energy (shorter wavelength) photons come into existence but that many of the low-energy (longer wavelength) photons are attenuated as successive HVLs are achieved. The practical value of half-value layers becomes apparent during the application of filtration.

FACTORS RELATING TO FILM DENSITY

The density of an x-ray film often is considered in relation to fundamental factors; e.g., kVp, mAs, FFD, object thickness, films and screens. While there is nothing wrong in these considerations they are not really all-encompassing. Other factors also play a part in determining film density. To reduce retake rates, thus keeping radiation dosages at a

Fog Reducers and Eliminators	Film Care and Handling Complete Film Protection from Ionizing Radiation Ideal Film Processing Procedures Optimal Grid (Ratio, Lines per cm/in) Type of Cassette
Density Producers	Intensity of kVp _____ mAs Value X-ray Apparatus and its efficiency Size, Type, Serviceability of Tube Target Electricity Intake (Supply) Line Film Speed Screen Speed
Density and Radiation Exposure Reducers	Added Filtration DEF (Density Equalizing Filtration) Increased FFD
Variables	Variations of: Object Size Object Density Area of Interest Field Size
Personal Preferences	Subjective Density Preference- Including Contrast Viewing Conditions-Including Type and Intensity of Light

minimum, it is reasonable to consider fully the factors pertaining to optimal film density when calculating the requirements of an x-ray exposure.

Chapter 2

The Point System of Exposure Calculation

On some modern generators, if all possible kV, mA, and the time settings are considered, the operator may select one of a possible 19,280 combinations! It would therefore seem practical to have some simplified method for selection of technique factors.

T. T. Thompson, *A Practical Approach to Modern X-ray Equipment*, p. 38, Little, Brown & Company, 1978.

The point system of exposure calculation was introduced by the Siemens organization in 1950. It has since proven to be one of the most accurate and reliable methods for preparing individual exposure charts, for recalculation of exposure data for different conditions, and in allowing for differing film speeds, screen speeds, grid retardations and supply line insufficiencies.

The following is a simplified explanation of the point system, presented in a limited form. For further information on this system, please refer to: "*EXPOSURE CALCULATIONS*, The Siemens Point System adapted for CHIROPRACTIC *SPINOGRAPHY*" by F. G. Bauer, or contact the Siemens Company directly.

To obtain a radiograph of optimum density two groups of exposure factors must be considered:

1. The mAs product and the focus-film distance;

2. The tube voltage and the thickness of the patient.

The radiation dose that passes through the patient and blackens the film is dependent upon the two groups above. This dose is directly proportional to the mAs and inversely proportional to the square of the focus-film distance. This dose is likewise proportional to the tube voltage and geometrically weakened by the patient's body. In most areas of the body the dose is reduced by each centimeter of tissue thickness. This logarithmic-based exposure system reveals that, on the average, each centimeter increase in tissue thickness calls **for an increase in the mAs product to a factor of 1.25. That is, one exposure point more requires 25 percent more dose or mAs product; three exposure points requires twice the mAs product.**

The advantage of this system is that all necessary calculations are carried out by

Figure 2-1
INITIAL EXPOSURE VALUES (IEV) FOR VARIOUS EXPOSURES OF THE SPINE WITH NORMAL OBJECT THICKNESS (NOT)

Vertebrae			IEV Points	NOT in cm
Cervical	1-7	A-P	24	13
"	1-7	Oblique	23	12
"	1-7	Lateral	22	11
Thoracic	1-4	A-P	26	15
"	5-12	A-P	30	22
"	2-4	Lateral	36	39
"	5-12	Lateral	30	30
Lumbar	1-5	A-P	30	22
"	1-5	Oblique	31	23
"	1-4	Lateral	35	31
Lumbo-Sac.	L5-S1	Lateral	37	33

simply adding or subtracting whole numbers, called points.

Basic exposure conditions have been arrived at for various areas of interest, and they are called Initial Exposure Values (a numerical point value). The Initial Exposure Values are calculated upon

1. normal object thickness (standard dimensions taken from the exposure tables by Janker, Mayer and Sakowsky);
2. 100 centimeter focus-film distance;
3. medium speed intensifying screens;
4. fast film;
5. without grid.

Figure 2-1 is a table providing the points assigned Initial Exposure Values (IEVs).

Where deviations from the norms as stated in the IEVs are encountered, exposure values must be corrected. For example, the IEV calls for a focus-film distance of 100 cm (40″). This distance should be altered to 200 cm (80″) for quality radiographic work. Thus, zero points are necessary for a 100 cm FFD exposure while an additional five points are required for a 185 cm (72″) FFD exposure and an additional six points for an exposure of 210cm (83″). Refer to Fig. 2-2

for a table of focus-film distance variations.

Grids are not allowed for in the IEV calculations. An 8:1 grid requires three points additional exposure; 10:1 requires five points; 12:1 requires six points and 16:1 grid necessitates the addition of seven points to the IEV for a particular imaging examination.

Insofar as films are concerned, the average par speed film requires a further two points to be added to the IEV.

Medium speed screens are valued at zero points. With average high-definition (fine detail) screens an additional three points exposure is necessary. For high speed screens subtract three points from the exposure requirements. However, it must be stated that the estimation for some calcium tungstate high-speed screens mandates the subtraction of four points.

As discussed earlier, alterations in the Normal Object Thickness (NOT — determined by measuring the thickness of the patient at the level of interest) necessitate one point be added or subtracted for each centimeter variation from the number stated under NOT.

Figure 2-2		EXPOSURE VALUES IN POINTS		
Focus Film			**Grid**	
Distance	**Points**		**Ratio**	**Points**
100cm	0		8:1	+4
110cm	+1		10:1	+5
125cm	+2		12:1	+6
140cm	+3		16.1	+7
160cm	+4			
180cm	+5			
200cm	+6			

Figure 2-3 illustrates the balance that must be obtained to produce the optimum radiographic result in any given situation. If the NOT is altered the mAs must be altered proportionately, providing that the kVp setting remains unchanged.

Figure 2-4 provides a table of kVp and mAs values.

Sufficient information is now available to allow illustration of this system via example.

Example No. 1 - Lateral Cervical :   12cm Thickness

Initial Exposure Value	=	22 points
Normal Object Thickness	=	+1 "
FFD 200cm	=	+6 "
High Definition Screens	=	+3 "
Par Speed Film	=	+2 "
Grid, 12:1	=	+6 "
Total		40 points required to produce optimum result
Tube Voltage 100 kVp	=	20 points
Tube Current 100 mAs	=	20 points
		40 points

The exposure is made from a distance of 200cm, at 100 kVp. The only variable factor is the mAs. Another illustration will aid in clarification.

Example No. 2 - Lateral Cervical :   10cm Thickness

Initial Exposure Value	=	22 points
Cervical Thickness 10cm	=	-1 "
FFD 200cm	=	+6 "
High Definition Screens	=	+3 "
Par Speed Film	=	+2 "

Grid, 12:1	=	+ 6 "
Total		38 points required to produce optimum result
Tube Voltage 100 kVp	=	20 points
Tube Current 64 mAs	=	18 points
		38 points

Example No. 2 is of a smaller individual than in the first instance. Still, all factors are unchanged except the mAs which is reduced from 100 mAs to 64 mAs. All that is necessary is to measure the patient with an accurate caliper and alter the mAs as required, leaving all other factors unchanged. This is the advantage of the Bauer adaptation of the point system for spinography: the distance and kVp are standardized so that the only altered machine setting is for the mAs, which depends on the measured thickness of the part to be examined. Once the x-ray user has prepared an exposure chart the point system is amazingly simple and effective to use. Various thicknesses are listed for each view taken and a corresponding mAs rating is prepared for each of these individual views. The kVp remains fixed at 100, the FFD remains fixed at 200cm (80"), the patient is measured at the level of interest and the thickness of the part determines what mAs setting is to be utilized.

Example No. 3 - Lateral Lumbar @ L5 Level : 33cms Thickness

Initial Exposure Value	=	37 points
Normal Object Thickness		
33cm	=	0 "
FFD 200cm	=	+6 "
High Speed Screens	=	-4 "
Par Speed Film	=	+2 "
Grid, 12:1	=	+6 "
Total		47 points required to produce optimum result
Tube Voltage 100 kVp	=	20 points
Tube Current 500 mAs	=	27 points
		47 points

Note that the only variable in the exposure setting between the cervical films and the lumbar film is the alteration in mAs. The kVp and FFD have remained unchanged. For the cervical and lumbar areas, obviously, different intensifying screens will be used, but it must be remembered that they too will be standardized to meet their respective requirements.

EXPOSURE REQUIREMENTS

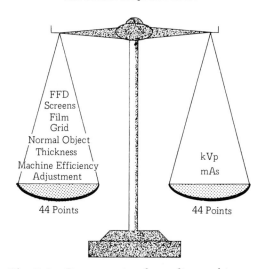

Fig. 2-3 - Components of a radiographic exposure must balance to produce the optimal final film result.

Example No. 4 - Lateral Lumbar @L5 Level:30cms

		Thickness
Initial Exposure Value	=	37 points
Lumbar Thickness 30cm	=	-3 "
FFD 200cm	=	+3 "
High Speed Screens	=	-4 "

Par Speed Film	=	+2 "
Grid, 12:1	=	+6 "
Total		44 points required to produce optimum result
Tube Voltage 100 kVp	=	20 points
Tube Current 250 mAs	=	24 points
		44 points

The patient thickness has decreased by only 3cm as compared to Example No. 3. However, the mAs has decreased by 50 percent.

It can readily be seen that the point system is a useful method of demonstrating the individual constituents which go to make up an x-ray exposure. It is an accurate way to calculate technique factors and to correct faulty exposures. With the help of this method a chart can be prepared to suit a wide range of x-ray machines.

Further particulars will assist the reader in understanding the refinements of this system.

Screens of apparently the same descriptive label — high definition, fast, etc. — can actually vary in speed by four points. It is essential to ascertain the speed of the particular screens before embarking on the preparation of an exposure table. Aged screens lose luminescence, which directly affects the outcome of any experiments.

When examining children from six to fourteen years of age, deduct one point from the total required to produce the optimum result.

For young adults, particularly males with better than average muscular development and substantial osseous structures, add one point.

With elderly patients with poor muscle tone and possible demineralization, deduct one point.

The Machine Efficiency Adjustment (MEA) must be heeded in preparing an

Figure 2-4

TABLE OF kVp & mAs POINTS

kVp Points		mAs Points		
40	= 0	1	=	0
41	= 1	1.25	=	1
42	= 2	1.6	=	2
44	= 3	2	=	3
46	= 4	2.5	=	4
48	= 5	3.2	=	5
50	= 6	4	=	6
52	= 7	5	=	7
55	= 8	6.4	=	8
57	= 9	8	=	9
60	= 10	10	=	10
63	= 11	12.5	=	11
66	= 12	16	=	12
70	= 13	20	=	13
73	= 14	25	=	14
77	= 15	32	=	15
81	= 16	40	=	16
85	= 17	50	=	17
90	= 18	64	=	18
96	= 19	80	=	19
102	= 20	100	=	20
109	= 21	125	=	21
117	= 22	160	=	22
125	= 23	200	=	23
		250	=	24
		320	=	25
		400	=	26
		500	=	27
		640	=	28
		800	=	29
		1000	=	30

exposure chart. It is quite likely that two high tension transformers of identical manufacture and model will vary in output. (Likewise, filament transformers can vary in output.) After all other considerations are reviewed and found to be of proper standard, a few trial films — preferably with a phantom — are in order. If the films are too dark, one or more points will have to be deducted to arrive at the correct density. If it is necessary to add exposure points, the installation should be inspected by a capable service representative. In considering the MEA a few areas of investigation may include: the line supply (line voltage), mAs and kVp output, tube focal spot and disc, the grid, its ratio and material for interspacing.

Processing of all films must be conducted precisely and with consistency or all attempts at standardization will prove fruitless. Using weakened developer could necessitate an additional three points exposure. An incorrect developing time would further jeopardize results.

The losses of luminescence which occur with older screens necessitate one or two points be added in calculating the factors for an exposure.

It must be remembered that, as far as tube efficiency and screen efficiencies are concerned, the point system of exposure calculation is based on new — or nearly new—equipment.

There is no magic answer to exposure charts. The seemingly eternal search for a simplified exposure system which functions at 100 percent accuracy 100 percent of the time is non-existent. There are too many variables for such a dream-land to exist. It takes consistent effort to produce consistently good radiographic results. The point system of exposure calculation is offered because it is reliable, it encompasses broad parameters of information input, it allows for systematic correction of technique inexactitude and it assists in the understanding of radiation subject matter. If the exposure system you now utilize is inadequate, and you have considered adopting an alternative method, the point system of exposure calculation may be of assistance.

Practical Perspective

COMPARISON OF IMAGING TECHNIQUES

LONG FFD (FSD)
Advantages:
1. Less Radiation
2. Less Distortion
3. Improved Definition
4. Less Magnification

HIGH kVp
Advantages:
1. Less Radiation
2. Good Penetration

LOW mAs
Advantages:
1. Less Radiation
2. Greater Tonal Range

SHORT FFD (FSD)
Disadvantages:
1. More Radiation
2. More Distortion
3. Reduced Definition
4. More Magnification

LOW kVp
Disadvantages:
1. More Radiation
2. Poor Penetration in Dense Area

HIGH mAs
Disadvantages:
1. More Radiation
2. Reduced Tonal Range

Chapter 3

X-Ray Tubes

In general, we should use radiation of the highest energy consistent with diagnostic quality x-ray films in order to minimize patient exposure.

E. E. Christensen, T. S. Curry, J. E. Dowdey, *An Introduction to the Physics of Diagnostic Radiology*, p. 53, 2nd Edition, Lea & Febiger, 1978.

Electrical energy is converted into **ionizing radiation within that rugged yet** delicate portion of radiographic equipment — the x-ray tube. Given care it will repay an x-ray user with several years of **trouble-free performance. But, should a** hapless operator execute one too many exposures within a brief time frame, he will be rewarded with the not insignificant expense of replacing the now useless x-ray tube.

X-ray tubes are wonders of modern science. So too are the generators that provide electrical power to the tubes. Before turning our attention to the study of x-ray tubes, a brief review of generators is appropriate.

Generators

Electrical power is necessary to activate an x-ray tube. This energy is supplied through the control console, the transformer and the rectifiers which serve the tube.

Modern generators are either single-phase or three-phase in electrical orientation. Rectification has been discussed and illustrated in the first chapter. Nearly all generators are now fully rectified; i.e., the alternating current of 60 cycles per second is rectified so that two pulses occur every 1/60 second, or 120 pulses per second. (With the 50-cycle-per second electrical power used in Australia, New Zealand and Europe there would be two pulses every 1/50 second or 100 pulses per second.) The single-phase, fully-rectified generator is the most common type used in conventional radiography.

Three-Phase Generators

The three-phase generator is becoming increasingly popular as the benefits of its more even output come to be appreciated. As illustrated in Fig. 3-1, three-phase supply involves an overlapping of cycles so that the electrical output remains nearly constant.

Three-phase generators are either six-pulse or twelve-pulse. In other words, six pulses or twelve pulses of electricity will occur during a normal cycle of 1/60 second. In the case of a single-phase unit the output varies from 0 percent to 100 percent twice during each cycle. This voltage differential is called the *ripple factor*, which is responsible for a lessened overall output of kilovoltage. Fig. 3-2 compares ripple factors and the increased strength of the three-phase generator can be readily appreciated. The ripple factor for six-pulse units is 13.5 percent and the corresponding figure for twelve-pulse equipment is 5 percent. The minimal ripple factor ensures a superior tube output.

Three Phase Alternating Current

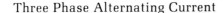
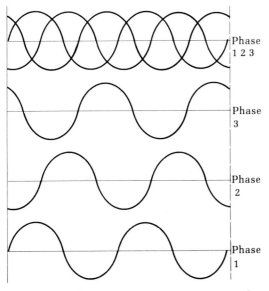

Fig. 3-1 — The output of three-phase current is superior to and more even than that of fully-rectified single-phase current.

In comparison to single-phase generators, three-phase generators produce more x-rays per cycle and the x-rays so produced are of higher average kilovoltage. Also, the anode is heated more evenly which allows the operator to make a larger exposure. At 100 kVp the ap-

proximate average kilovoltage from a single-phase generator is 70 kV while the corresponding kilovoltage for a three-phase, six-pulse generator is 95 kV and for three-phase, twelve-pulse equipment, 98 kV. The rise in popularity of three-phase units is readily understood when one considers their advantages.

Capacitor discharge generators store electrical power within a complex capacitor arrangement, the exposure taking place within several millionths of a second as the energy is released to the tube. The present level of technology of capacitor discharge units renders them acceptable for small body part exposures. However, they are inadequate for the heavy demands of spinal imaging procedures.

Generator Capacity & Choice of Equipment

The capacity of a generator/tube combination is an important consideration. Advertisements will declare that a particular piece of equipment is a "300/125 unit" or a "500/150 unit." The unsuspecting reader may believe that the machines produce 300 mA at 125 kVp and 500 mA at 150 kVp, respectively. Perhaps they will — for a few milliseconds. The maximum kilovoltage and milliampere ratings do not usually function concurrently.

How does the foregoing relate to the practical matter of purchasing a suitable x-ray unit? Advertising claims notwithstanding, such variables as peaky waveform patterns, current losses through filament transformer and autotransformer, less-than-ideal primary electricity supply and voltage fluctuations from daily and seasonal load variations render the selection of suitable equipment an adventure for the gullible or unwary.

The only certain way to determine machine effectiveness is to view radiographs taken by the apparatus in question. Excellence in spinal radiography requires a unit capable of producing a highly diagnostic film of the fifth lumbar area in the lateral position from a distance of 150-

200cms (60-80"). As a guide to the mettle of an x-ray machine, it can be stated that the equipment should be able to function at 100 kVp for 600 mAs or at 125 kVp for 320 mAs.

It is appropriate to delve deeper into the matter of equipment selection. In an excellent book by Thomas T. Thompson, *A Practical Approach to Modern X-Ray Equipment* (Little, Brown & Co., 1978) he states with regard to choosing a unit —

> *"Service should be the most important consideration in deciding what brand of radiographic equipment is to be purchased."*

There is more value in that single sentence than some roentgenology texts encompass between front and back covers. Until one has waited two days with an installation experiencing "down time," the concept of service may not seem all that important. A conscientious, capable and reliable service department

RIPPLE FACTORS

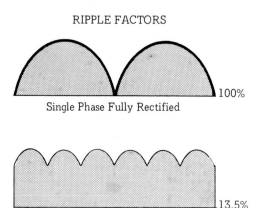

Single Phase Fully Rectified — 100%

Three Phase 6-Pulse — 13.5%

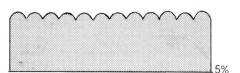

Three Phase 12-Pulse — 5%

Fig. 3-2 — Although the largest percentage of conventional diagnostic x-ray units are single-phase, fully-rectified models, the three-phase, twelve-pulse models produce the most efficient wave-form.

is a real boon to the busy x-ray facility. Talk to associates and ascertain the reputation of various x-ray firms in your locale. An organization without a reputation for integrity should be shunned.

X-ray Tubes

An x-ray tube consists of two electrodes — the cathode and the anode —installed within a vacuum and allowing electrical current to flow in one direction. The tungsten filament of the cathode is heated to the point where excited electrons escape from the metal via *thermionic emission*. The electrons hovering about the filament comprise the *space charge*. This "cloud" of electrons can be drawn to the anode by the application of an electric current. The negatively-charged electrons leave the cathode to collide with the positively-charged anode and produce x-ray radiation. X-ray production is as inefficient as are many of our present level-of-knowledge technologies: approximately 99 percent of energy expenditure results in the production of heat while only one percent of the reactive process yields x-rays.

Because of the magnitude of heat production the anode must be treated with well-deserved respect. Let us outline the path of some just-propagated x-ray photons as they leave the anode. If the radiation is not attenuated within the tube itself, it will traverse the tube port, bridge the glass envelope of the tube, and pass through the mantle of oil which assists tube cooling. The photons should now be intercepted by an aluminum filter 2mm thick.

This filtration removes many of the longer-wavelength, "softer" rays which lack the penetrating power to pass through the filter material. The beam is now relatively "hardened" because a greater proportion of shorter-wavelength rays remain. The stream of photons enters the collimator where the mirror arrests a small number of x-rays and the lead shutters intercept all rays which are

ROTATING ANODE X-RAY TUBE

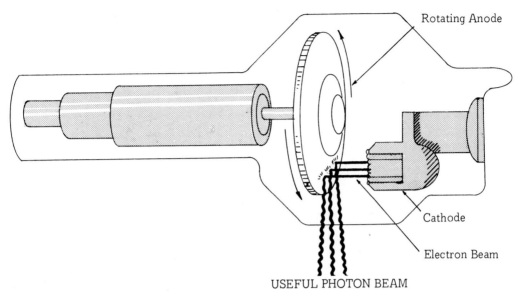

Rotating Anode

Cathode

Electron Beam

USEFUL PHOTON BEAM

Fig. 3-3 — The rotating anode tube is a "must" for today's vertebral imaging system.

not directed at the useful area of the film. The collimator has pared the original cone-shaped beam into a rectangular configuration which comprises an arc of very few degrees at the recommended focus-film distance of 200cm (80″).

If density equalizing filtration located in front of the collimator is used, the beam is attenuated once again. Most of the remaining photons proceed through the expanse of air until they reach the patient. After the patient has been penetrated, the remnant beam has to proceed through the bucky front, the grid and the cassette front to finally arrive at the intensifying screens and the film emulsion.

It really is quite astonishing to realize that a diagnostic quality image can be produced after such a thorough depletion of energy has taken place. The anode is vitally important to the production of a diagnostic radiograph, as this brief account illustrates. It is no wonder that a damaged anode reduces the "picture-taking capabilities" of an x-ray machine to such a marked degree.

Anatomy & Physiology of an X-Ray Tube

Spinal imaging requisites dictate the need for a rotating anode tube; the stationary anode tube has a limited loading capacity and is more suitable for exposing a hand or a foot than a portion of the vertebral column or pelvis. The rotating anode tube, Fig. 3-3, was first proposed by a French author prior to 1900 and only went into effective production during the 1920's. During the past 50 years improvements in rotating anode tubes have occurred but the basic principles concerning their function remain unchanged.

The rotating anode consists of an anode disc and a rotor body, or shaft, which is responsible for the rotation of the disc. The anode disc is made of tungsten or a tungsten alloy and the surface usually is tungsten with a small amount of rhenium added. Tungsten provides an adequate source of x-rays, but if used solely it allows a rapid roughening of the target area to occur. As soon as a tube is "run in" surface imperfections will appear on the focal track. At this stage the disc surface should resemble fine sandpaper in ap-

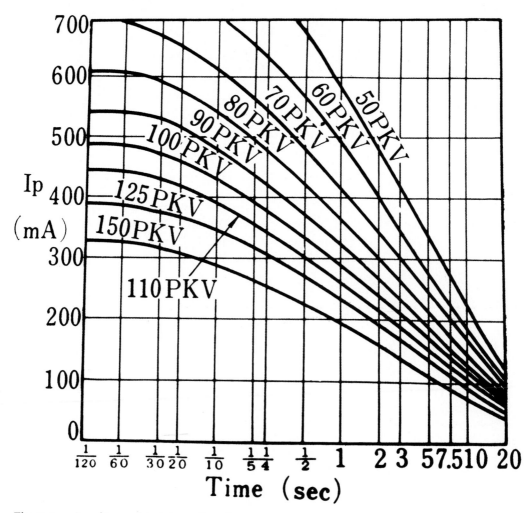

Fig. 3-4 — A radiographic tube rating chart.

pearance. Normally this does not affect the production of x-rays which are generated consistently for years (with due care). At such time as severe roughening does occur, the yield of x-rays drops precipitously and the effective life of the tube usually ends shortly thereafter.

The typical anode diameter varies from 75 to 125mm and the anode rotates at a theoretical 3,600 RPM (60 cycles per second, 60 seconds per minute). In Australia, New Zealand and Europe on 50 cps current the theoretical anode rotation rate is 3,000 RPM (50 cycles per second, 60 seconds per minute). Mechanical factors prevent anodes from attaining their theoretical speeds; nevertheless, under normal operating conditions anode speeds are such that the resulting heat buildup is satisfactorily dissipated.

The anode stem is made of molybdenum which has a high melting point and low heat conductivity. Rotating anode tubes cool by radiation and thus the stem aids in preventing excess heat from reaching the bearings located behind it.

The bearings operate within a vacuum where standard lubricants become unstable and form a gas. This gaseous product of chemical instability will diminish the vacuum to the point where the tube is no longer functional.

Electrons are supplied to the anode by the cathode. The cathode in most modern

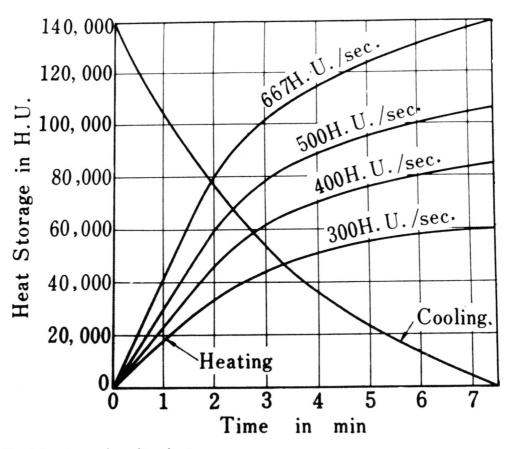

Fig. 3-5 — An anode cooling chart.

tubes contains a *focusing cup* which houses two filaments. One filament is for smaller exposures and it obtains finer details acting through the small focal spot. The larger filament and larger focal spot withstand higher exposures but there is a reduction of radiographic detail. The anode and cathode assemblies are housed within a *glass envelope* which is commonly made of Pyrex. This entity is known as the *tube insert*. When a tube fails, service personnel may replace the entire tube structure although most often replacement of the tube insert is all that is required. Of course the cost of supplying a new tube is substantially more than the cost of a new tube insert.

As tubes age the glass wall assumes a "sunburnt" appearance, a gradually deepening bronzing. This is a tungsten coating which forms on the glass, mostly from the filament but lesser amounts stemming from the anode. If the filament is operated at high temperatures for large mA exposures, tungsten begins to evaporate. This vaporization does not occur immediately but progresses the longer the filament is maintained at a high temperature.

The important fact to be learned from the above is that holding the "prep" button in an active state for lengthy periods harms the x-ray tube. Modern tubes are ready to be activated within one second; keeping the tube "boosted" for ten seconds means that the excessive preparation time is causing filament evaporation. Continued repeatedly this fault could actually bring about the tube's destruction.

Like automobiles and airplanes, television and trouser zippers, a rotating anode tube eventually wears out. The target becomes too pitted from the heat of too many high-speed electron bombardments and simply gives up the ghost. Just so this matter is kept in perspective, remember that there have been tubes known to have taken over one million small exposures, all because the anode material never became too hot.

Anode Heel Effect

The intensity of radiation is not even across the entire beam. There is a fall-off in intensity on the anode side of the beam which is known as the *anode heel effect*. This phenomenon occurs because photons emerging from a beveled focal track on the anode face must pass through more metal than photons more perpendicularly directed; i.e., at the cathode side of the tube. Angles close to those of the anode face suffer more attenuation or filtration of radiation.

If, for example, an A-P Thoracic visualization is contemplated from an FFD of 40 inches, the tube should be aligned so that the cathode end of the beam is directed at a lower thoracic vertebrae. The upper thoracic region is more easily penetrated and should receive the anode portion of the beam.

The anode heel effect is almost of historical interest when discussing modern imaging techniques. The longer focus-film distances of 150cm (60″), and especially 200cm (80″), decrease the heel effect to a point where it is no longer diagnostically useful or even particularly significant.

Tube Rating & Cooling Charts

When creating x-rays excessive heat can be produced in a very short time. Manufacturers are well aware of this fact and they issue a rating chart similar to the example shown in Fig. 3-4 for each of the tubes in their range. Rating charts apply to specific tubes; they are not interchangeable among various models or firms. The tube rating chart will vary according to the size of the focal-spot, the

rectification and the anode's speed, diameter and angle. The chart will inform the reader of the maximum mA, kV and exposure time which can be used for a particular exposure. Because most modern generators are equipped with automatic overload protection which renders units inoperable if a single exposure exceeds the maximum tube rating, many people believe that tube rating charts are of academic interest only. This definitely is not the case. There is no switch, overload protection or other fail-safe mechanism which prevents an individual from pressing the exposure button too soon after the previous exposure. Conducting three examinations of the lumbar spine in quick succession has definite potential for causing great harm to an x-ray tube. If two exposures of maximum rating are executed, the second occurring before the anode has had time to cool sufficiently (maximum heat rating plus retained heat), damage to the anode can be expected.

How much heat has been generated and how long it will take for this heat to dissipate is plotted on an anode cooling chart, a representative example of which is illustrated in Fig. 3-5. One fallacy in referring to anode cooling charts pertains to the "baseline" reading at the time the chart is read. The mantle of oil which surrounds the tube is assumed to be at room temperature any time the chart is consulted. This is only true for the first exposure within a specific time period. Exposures following shortly thereafter cannot be treated in the same way since the oil mantle has been warmed and it now offers lessened cooling qualities. It is reasonable to allow adequate cooling periods after an exposure or a series of exposures has been conducted; it is unreasonable to have to replace a tube destroyed by excessive heat.

Heat Units

The quantity of heat deposited within an x-ray tube is measured in *heat units* (HU). The heat unit value is a product of kilovoltage, milliamperage and time:

Heat Units = kVp x mA x seconds
An exposure of 100 kVp and 200 mAs produces 20,000 HU

100 kVp x 200 mA x 1 sec = 20,000 HU

70 kVp x 1,000 mAs = 43 points = 70,000 HU
100 kVp x 200 mAs = 43 points = 20,000 HU

The formula stated above applies to single-phase equipment. Three-phase equipment utilizes the same formula plus a correction factor of 1.35 which is multiplied to the final product because of its near constant output. The example illustrated above would yield 27,500 HUs if produced on three-phase equipment.

We advocate a high-optimal kilovoltage technique as being the safest method for patients from the radiation point of view. It is interesting to note that a high-optimal kilovoltage technique is also kind to x-ray tubes. Let us consider two exposures of 43 points each, according to the point system of exposure calculation. As long as the points are equal, each exposure will produce the same film density. Examine the heat units produced in each of the following examples:

Not only does the patient receive less radiation with high-optimal kilovoltage technique but the tube receives considerable benefit from the reduced heat unit burden.

Exceeding the limits of heat units allowed in manufacturers' charts can cause immediate roughening of the focal track or, if the abuse is severe enough, melting of the anode. The oil mantle may be heated beyond its ability to recover, permitting the entire tube to perish. Repeated exposures with inadequate cooling times can warp an anode while a single heavy exposure to a cold anode can cause that anode to crack. It is always a good idea to "warm" an anode before embarking upon the day's first examination procedure. An exposure of 40 kVp at 100 mA for 0.2 seconds produces only 800 HU but this could well extend the life of the tube.

Practical Perspective

TESTING AN X-RAY TIMER

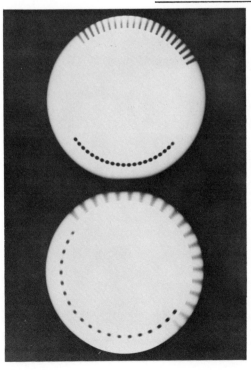
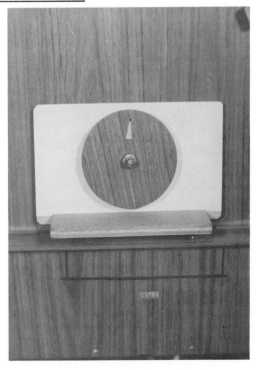

If the timing mechanism of an x-ray machine is not performing accurately, the radiographic result will be improperly exposed films. A simple way to check the timer is with a "spinning top." A metal disc, usually made of brass or lead, is placed in front of a loaded cassette. The spinning top has a notch or a hole in it so that when the disc is rotated during a test exposure the accuracy of the timer can be determined.

The output of a single-phase fully-rectified generator occurs in pulses, not in a continuous stream. If the output was constant the spinning top would produce a solid line during the time of the exposure. Sixty cycles per second current yields 120 pulses every second with full rectification. An exposure lasting one-tenth of a second would produce 12 dashes on the film with a spinning top if the timer functioned accurately. A one-fifth second exposure would produce 24 pulses. However, care must be taken when spinning the top to ensure that it does not travel a complete circle during the test exposure.

The radiograph illustrated in this example was exposed in Australia where the current is 50 cycles per second. Full rectification yields 100 current pulses per second. The timer was set for one-fifth second, which produces 20 current pulses when the mechanism operates accurately. Twenty-one current pulses occurred in the upper illustration, revealing that the time functioned slightly in error.

Practical Perspective

DAMAGED ANODES

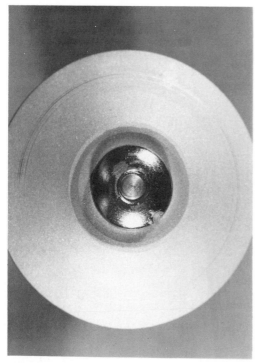 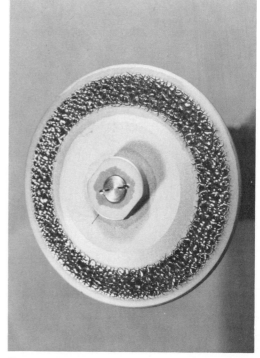

A   B

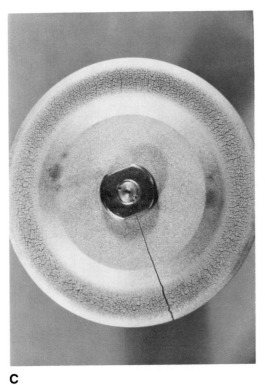

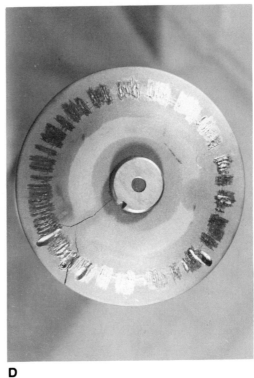

C **D**

The rotating anode shown in (A) is essentially normal. The focal track is observable and undamaged. The anode in (B) is so heavily crazed along the path of the focal track that x-ray output would be minimal. A simple yet complete crack extends through the radius of anode (C). Anode (D) is the most interesting specimen. Not only is the anode cracked, it has multiple areas of focal track damage. Faulty operation has allowed electron bombardment to hit a non-moving anode, each "hit" overheating and thus marring a portion of the anode surface.

Chapter 4

Grid System

Radiologists know, yet few clinicians appreciate, that almost every radiographic examination is a compromise. More information may be obtained by the use of additional exposures, detail grids or slow film — but at the expense of a higher radiation dose.

C. S. Houston, M. H. Shokeir, *Potential Hazards of Diagnostic Radiation*, 28:62-68, p. 62, Journal of the Canadian Association of Radiologists, 1977.

Scattered radiation is probably the single most important factor leading to poor diagnostic quality films. The fog produced by scatter radiation reduces contrast and definition, causing film blackening from the scattered rays which leave the patient in all directions.

In 1913 Dr. Gustave Bucky invented the first x-ray grid. A grid is an arrangement of thin lead strips which are interspaced with a translucent material. The purpose of the grid is to remove secondary radiation and to allow only those photons which originate at the focal spot to pass in a straight line to reach the film, as shown in Fig. 4-1. The grid is located between the patient and the film so that scatter radiation arising from the patient is "filtered" out of the final film result as well. Fig 4-1 B depicts primary radiation traveling straight through the interspacing material to reach the film while scatter radiation is being "cleaned-up" by the lead strips of the grid.

Just seven years after Bucky's invention, Dr. Potter developed the moving grid which became known as the Potter-Bucky diaphragm. Today the Potter-Bucky diaphragm is referred to simply as "the bucky." The stationary grid is more economical and is easier to fix in a completely motionless position. However, the visible grid lines may be distracting at normal viewing distances.

Grids are either focused or parallel in design. More x-rays are attenuated at the edge of the film than at the center with a finite-focused parallel grid. Consequently, in diagnostic roentgenography the focused linear grid receives by far the greatest acceptance. The grid cutoff referred to above happens in a parallel grid as the lead strips intercept primary photons toward the edges of an x-ray beam. With a focused grid, cutoff may also occur if the grid is used at an

SCHEMATIC ILLUSTRATION OF GRID EFFECT

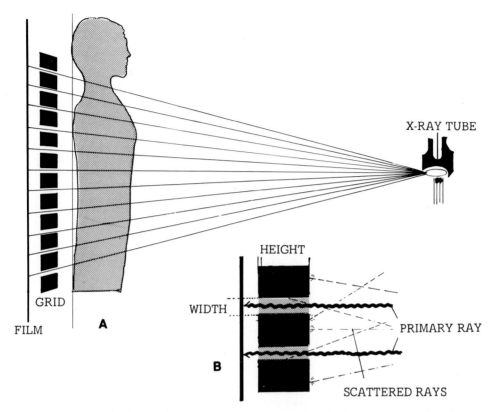

Fig. 4-1 — A grid allows photons passing in a straight line from the focal spot to reach the film. The insert shows how scattered photons are prevented from reaching the film by the lead strips.

improper distance from its point of focus. The manufacturer often indicates how much distance deviation from the correct focus distance is permissible. If this distance is not known a general rule states that all exposures should be made within ten percent of the grid focus distance. Fig. 4-2 illustrates off-distance cutoff, off-center cutoff and off-level cutoff, all three problems arising from incorrect installation or use of focused grids. Off-distance cutoff occurs when a grid is used at a distance incompatible with the focusing range of that grid. Off-center cutoff occurs when the grid is laterally decentered in relation to the focal spot of the tube. A uniformly pale x-ray film results and this fault may be blamed incorrectly on errors in exposure technique. Off-level cutoff takes place when the grid is tilted in relation to its normal perpendicular alignment to the central ray. It also brings about a lessened overall film density. A focused grid yields an x-ray picture of even density from edge to edge, assuming of course that it is properly centered and leveled.

A grid which is focused at 100cm (40") is completely unsuitable for use at 180cm (72"). With a stationary grid great care should be taken to ensure that the central ray is maintained at right angles to the center of the grid. With a moving grid, the central ray should be at a right angle to the center of the grid exactly at the midpoint of the grid's travel. Unless this

THREE COMMON FORMS OF GRID CUTOFF

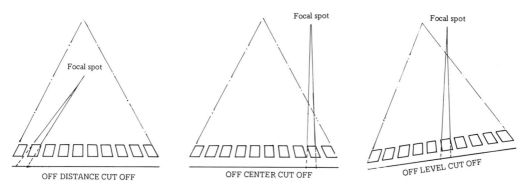

Fig. 4-2 — A focused grid will "cut off" primary rays if it is positioned at an incorrect distance, if it is not centered accurately or if it is not perpendicular to the central ray.

factor is considered, primary rays may be attenuated on one side or the other. When placing a grid in position care must be taken to ensure that the grid focus is indeed where the anode is expected to be during operation; otherwise useful primary rays will be cut off. For purposes of information and installation a conspicuous line is often located on one side of a grid by the manufacturer. The side with this line must face the x-ray tube, installed so that the line is vertical. Other manufacturers omit this line and include a printed sticker which carries the "Tube Side" message.

Grid Ratio

Grid ratio is a term used in describing the functional capacity of a grid. The grid ratio is the height of the lead strips divided by the distance between the strips. (Refer back to Fig. 4-1 B for an illustration of the grid ratio.) Expressed by an equation the formula is:

$$\text{Grid Ratio} = \frac{\text{height of grid strips}}{\text{distance between grid strips}}$$

$$R = \frac{h}{d}$$

In early days of grid usage a 2:1 grid would have been common. This means that the distance from the tube side of the grid to the film side of the grid is twice the size of each of the spaces between the

lead strips. Remember, the thickness of the lead strips is not a factor in the calculation of a grid's ratio. Today grids are 8:1, 10:1 and more. In fact, no x-ray installation working with 100 kVp and above should have less than a 12:1 grid; this point will be explained further on in this chapter.

The illustration in Fig. 4-3 shows exactly why a 16:1 grid is so much more effective than is an 8:1 grid in removing scatter radiation. The maximum angle at which secondary radiation will pass through the grid is 7° in an 8:1 grid, 5.25° in a 12:1 grid and 3.5° in a 16:1 grid.

In addition to the grid ratio, a further descriptive label applied to a grid relates to the number of lead strips per unit of distance. A grid may be labeled "10:1/85 L.P.I." This means that there are 85 lines per inch of grid surface. Metric countries label their grids in centimeters. For example, a grid might be described as 10:1/40. This means that there are 40 lines per centimeter, or 103 lines per inch.

The lines-per-inch play an important role in scatter clean-up capabilities. A 12:1/85 L.P.I. grid will not be as efficient as a 12:1/103 L.P.I. grid manufactured by the same company.

The material used for the interspacers also bears upon the final outcome of the roentgenographic result. Early models contained wooden interspacers while today's grids utilize fiber, plastic or metal interspacers. By far the best interspacer material is aluminum. Aluminum is quite effective because it cleans up a portion of the well-aligned scatter radiation which, because of its parallel orientation, escapes the lead strips that have held back other scattered rays.

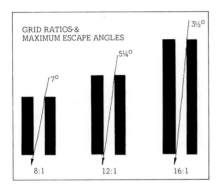

Fig. 4-3 — As grid ratios increase, the maximum escape angles for scattered radiation progressively decrease.

Of course there is a practical limit beyond which attenuation will affect diagnostic quality. This limit is generally governed by the tube tension — kVp. At 100 kVp perhaps the best all-round grid is 12:1/103 L.P.I. with aluminum interspacers. This was the conclusion reached after testing 45 different grids with other factors remaining unchanged. For spinal imaging requisites, at 120 kVp a 16:1 grid will prove more effective.

When using an x-ray machine whereby a minus adjustment has to be made for "machine efficiency adjustment," as per the point system, a 16:1 grid may be appropriate. If an efficient machine also has minimal intake line impedance, the 16:1 grid is highly recommended. Good electrical power factors are present more often in urban areas and so a 12:1 ratio grid may prove best for x-ray users in less than ideal rural situations.

In the construction of grids, lead strips are laid down in alternate steps with the interspacer material. This used to be a rather bulky, cumbersome task. However, technological developments have allowed grid construction to advance markedly. With present manufacturing methods, the thickness of lead strips varies from 0.0381mm to 0.889mm, i.e., 1.5- to 3.5 thousandths of an inch. When grids are tested for quality, the fine white lines represent shadows of the end-on view of the lead strips. These fine lines appear deceptively broad because of the crystal size in the film. If intensifying screens also are used, an entirely erroneous impression of the thickness of the grid strips is perceived, even if all the lead strips are focused exactly in line with the focal spot. The size of the tube's focal spot also aids in creating an illusionary impression of extra thickness in the lines.

The Orthogonal (crosshatch) crossed grid and the Rhombic crossed grid are two further varieties of grids sometimes used. Their acceptance has been restricted by increased tube current requirements as compared to linear grids. In addition, there are greater alignment difficulties with crossed grids, i.e., cephalad and caudal tube inclinations are prohibited. Rhombic or crosshatch grids are not economical with 100 kVp or less; excessive primary ray clean up occurs with their use.

If a 70 kVp technique has been in use for certain exposures and a change to 100 kVp is contemplated, a problem could well arise in regard to grid function. If, for example, an 8:1 grid is installed in the x-ray facility it would prove to be sadly lacking in clean up capabilities when used at the 100 kVp level. A 12:1 grid is necessary to clean up 100 kVp. Remember that a rising grid ratio is accompanied by an increased ability to filter scatter radiation and an increased exposure requirement to produce the optimum radiographic image. Therefore, a changeover to more powerful generating apparatus usually requires moving up to a higher ratio grid.

Lengthy experimentation has led us to reject commonly accepted recommendations pertaining to grid ratios and kVp settings. For example, 8:1 ratio grids have been advocated for use with exposure techniques up to a maximum of 100 kVp. In actual fact an 8:1 grid in conjunction with an exposure technique of 100 kVp is doomed to failure: an 8:1 grid successfully cleans up no more than 80 kVp.

The following list provides an accurate assessment of kilovoltages which may be used with various ratio grids.

Grid Ratio	Sufficient Up To — kVp
4:1	55
6:1	65
8:1	80
10:1	90
12:1	100
16:1	125
8:1 crosshatch	150

Reducing scatter radiation with a grid requires additional power to obtain a satisfactory film. The amount of additional power required varies with the grid ratio.

Grid Ratio	Additional Exposure "Points" Required	Percentage Increase In Power Required
8:1	4 Points	250%
10:1	5 "	320%
12:1	6 "	400%
16:1	7 "	500%
8:1 crosshatch	8 "	640%

All grids improve radiographic contrast. However, at higher kilovoltage settings a grid is not as effective as at lower kilovoltages. The main factor in this change relates to the effective absorption coefficient of the subject. As a general rule, the absorption coefficient lessens with increased kVp; above 100 kVp the subject contrast will decrease to a perceptible degree.

Lateral lumbar exposures are often responsible for the creation of prodigious amounts of scatter radiation (although, for accuracy's sake, it must be mentioned that to some extent the patient's own body assists in cleaning up a portion of the scatter rays in this view). Tests reveal that a good quality 16:1 grid, when used for a lateral lumbar exposure at 100 kVp, permits scatter to contribute 48 per cent of the film's blackening. The same grid at 125 kVp permits 60 percent blackening from scatter radiation sources.

A good grid is necessary to produce a good spinographic film; a poor grid simply allows for the creation of a poor film. More x-ray exposure is required with high-ratio grids but better contrast results. To ensure that the grid system does not contribute excessive radiation to the patient, it should be installed and maintained in peak operating order. A final recommendation is for a high grid ratio (12:1) in conjuction with high optimal kilovoltage; the patient does receive less radiation from this practice.

The Bucky

The name "bucky" is used often to refer to the grid alone whereas in actuality it entails the whole drive mechanism plus grid. It is this complete apparatus to which we now direct our attention.

The use of a bucky improves the viewing quality of any film. The white lines produced with a stationary grid are entirely absent with a properly functioning bucky. A fine line grid of, for example, 103 L.P.I. or more supposedly creates such narrow lines that they "dissolve" when films are read from the normal viewing distance of 30cm. Nevertheless, keen observers are unsettled by the presence of grid lines which divide the viewing area into as many segments as there are lead strips on the grid. A stationary grid undoubtedly affects the discernment of fine details and does provide an interruption within the viewing area. The fewer lead strips per inch, the more conspicuous they will be. Where spinal biomechanics are of concern the bucky will be mounted in an erect position. The upright bucky is supported by a bucky stand. This bucky stand should be constructed so that the bucky is perfectly steady and unvarying in its position during operation. It is of utmost importance that the bucky be maintained in a micro-steady state during all exposures.

Allowing bucky "shake" is one of the cardinal faults in diagnostic radiology. Bucky shake produces films of mediocre quality, particularly lacking in definition.

The film grain size varies from 1 to 1½ microns (1/1000 - 1.5/1000mm) across and the crystals of intensifying screens are 5 to 10 microns (5/1000 - 10/1000mm) in diameter. These crystals purportedly play a role in film definition — sharpness, resolution — and this role is not denied. However, should the bucky shake as little as 1 to 1.5 microns the benefits of a fine grain film are completely annihilated. And, should the bucky shake only 5 to 10 microns the definition of the intensifying screens also is destroyed. During inspections of x-ray installations, bucky wobbles of 1mm, 2mm and more have been detected. It is not necessary to have a great imagination to realize what harm can befall film quality through such bucky movement.

Poorly constructed bucky support and lack of maintenance to same are prime causes of unwanted bucky movement. The paraphrasing of an earlier admonition is worthwhile: A bucky must be micro-steady during operation if quality films are to be produced.

The three most common types of buckys are named by the mode of transport for the grid:
(1) Single Stroke
(2) Recipromatic
(3) Oscillating
Often the single stroke bucky is described further by being termed a single stroke catapult bucky. Upon activation the bucky mechanism initiates movement of the grid, which begins just before the exposure proper, completing its journey just after the exposure is finished. The particular period of extra movement is ideally 0.8 seconds before and after exposure. This precludes cutoff on either side, or what sometimes is labeled "false heel effect."

The single stroke bucky is activated by the release of a cog which is connected to a cylinder in the bucky's mechanism. This oil cylinder contributes to a smoothly operating bucky, providing that it is maintained in good working order. A specific lubricant is necessary to keep the cylinder functioning properly. The inadvertent supply of a heavier, greasier lubricant will cause operational difficulties in the bucky. Periodic inspection of the bucky mechanism, including oiling and honing of the release cog if indicated, is recommended as a preventative maintenance measure.

All this attention to detail is aimed at lessening any possible bucky frame movement. If, after careful scrutiny of the bucky mechanism, detectable movement persists, one must turn to the bucky stand and framework supporting the bucky

Catapult buckys are being phased out in favor of fresh designs. Nevertheless as long as it is well maintained a quality single stroke bucky can perform its task as well as newer models.

As the name indicates, a recipromatic bucky travels back and forth in front of the film plane. Recipromatic buckys are available in various speeds, the par speed model being quite suitable for spinographic studies where exposure times are not critically short.

An oscillating bucky acts as its name suggests, seemingly vibrating or quivering to prevent grid lines from appearing. This type of bucky is of less complex construction than the recipromatic bucky but it is quite capable of doing a thorough job of cleaning up scatter radiation. The bucky must be of particularly solid construction to prevent any movement of an oscillating grid from giving rise to unsharpness.

Stroboscopic Effect

A phenomenon known as *stroboscopic effect* can occur which results in the appearance of grid lines on the film. With single-phase, fully rectified two pulse circuits, 60 cycles yields 120 current pulses per second. It is possible for the current pulses to occur at exactly the same time that the lead strips of the grid are in line at a given spot on the film. When grid lines and current pulses coincide, white lines appear on the processed film because no radiation reached the film at these locations.

A common movie imperfection will explain the stroboscopic effect in practical terms. A spoked wagon in a western film will appear to be moving forward with fixed wheels when the frames of the film catch the spokes in the same position. If the frames are out of phase just slightly the wagon even appears to be moving forward with wheels that are turning backwards.

Sometimes this problem can be eliminated in catapult buckys by simply side-shifting the grid a minute amount within the bucky. In other instances a replacement grid with a different lines-per-inch value is unavoidable.

If stroboscopic effect occurs with a single stroke catapult bucky, and this is more likely at minimal exposures such as 0.1 or 0.2 seconds, corrective measures can often be accomplished by the individual x-ray user. Adjustment of tension in one of the two tension springs alters the speed of grid travel and frequently suffices to prevent stroboscopic effect. Consequently an adjustment of the timing knob is necessary.

System Performance

Grid lines may result from one or more of several diverse causes. The grid may fail to move upon actuation; the grid may move at an uneven speed; grid travel time may be excessive; the exposure may start before the grid is activated or continue after the grid has ceased motion; the tube may be situated in an off-center position relative to the grid. Each of these instances has a common thread running through its fabric: if the grid system is not up to standard the diagnostic quality of all films will be compromised.

The following prerequisites are essential for satisfactory grid-bucky performance:

(1) The bucky must be level so that cassettes will be stationed in a level manner;
(2) the floor beneath the bucky must be level;
(3) the bucky must face the central ray at an angle of 90°. Anything other than a right angle will result in cutoff;
(4) the tube must be positioned so that the bucky operates within the focal range of its enclosed grid;
(5) the bucky must not shake or wobble. It must be "micro-steady."

A builders' level is an apt tool for checking the alignment of the floor and the grid system mechanism. It is even edifying to go over the tube stand for alignment faults. In upright, bio-mechanically oriented diagnostic studies, it is obvious that any deficiency which results in the film being inferior on one side will likewise result in the patient appearing to be inferior on the same side.

Practical Perspective —

TESTING STABILITY OF EQUIPMENT

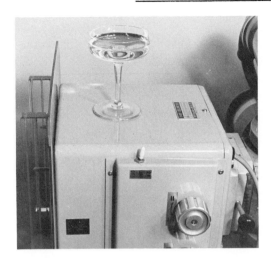

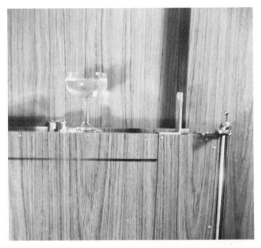

A   B

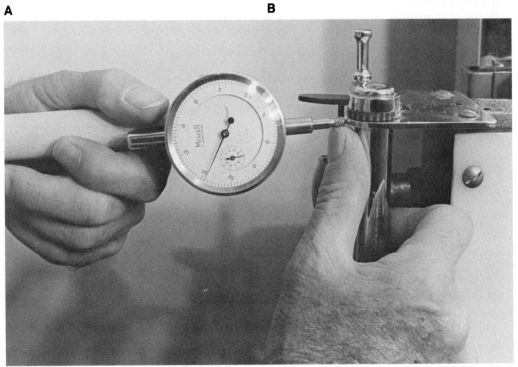

C

Movement of the patient during an imaging examination creates unsharpness in the final film result. Unwanted movement of the tube or the film also creates unsharpness. An anode rotates and a grid moves in front of the film surface but in neither instance should objectionable or unnecessary movement be permitted. There are simple, inexpensive ways to test the stability of x-ray equipment.

Perhaps the easiest method to determine if movement is originating in the tube involves the use of a shallow glass — or saucer — of water. Place the filled container upon the collimator and then activate the x-ray tube. If operation of the tube causes the appearance of ripples on the water, movement is occurring. Locating the glass on the collimator is worth noting. Because the collimator is attached to the tube which is attached to the tube stand, any movement which may occur close to the tube stand will be amplified—and more readily detected—at the end of the arc movement, i.e., the collimator.

The glass is next placed on top of the vertical bucky. When the bucky mechanism is activated no ripples should form. If ripples are visible it means that the film is experiencing this same movement, to the detriment of the final film result. The authors once tested a bucky which engendered such "bucky shake" that drops of water were thrown out of the glass. Interpretation of films taken in conjunction with this grid system should best be done by a fertile, inventive mind.

Another method of testing bucky stability is with the aid of a microdial. The microdial is installed between the bucky and a nearby wall, given support and snugly settled into position. When the bucky is activated the amount of bucky shake can be measured in "thou."

For the sharpest possible definition, all relevant imaging components must be kept micro-steady.

Chapter **5**

Film and Its Protection

Apart from the natural background, the main source of human exposure to ionizing radiation in the developed countries, results from diagnostic medical irradiations. The magnitudes of the individual doses delivered, and the large proportion of population exposed, suggest strongly that exposures can and should be substantially reduced, and that risk-benefit assessments be performed for several diagnostic procedures.

M. Disendorf, Editor, The Magic Bullet, Social Implications and Limitations of Modern Medicine, an Environmental Approach, p. 117, Society for Social Responsibility in Science (Australian Capital Territory), 1976.

From the time that an individual sheet of x-ray film leaves the factory until it is situated in a view box it may undergo any of approximately three hundred different mistakes. One lesser mistake can make an average film unacceptable. One fundamental mistake can reduce an otherwise superior film to the level of mediocrity.

Great care must be taken when dealing with radiographic film at all times. It does no good to utilize density-equalizing filtration if static marks from careless handling necessitate retake exposures.

Anatomy & Physiology of Radiographic Film

Modern x-ray film (Fig. 5-1) begins with a base layer most often composed of a polyester resin. The base is required to have dimensional stability, resistance to tearing, easy handling characteristics and appropriate flexibility. Its 0.15-0.02mm thickness often carries a blue tint which is optically more acceptable than the colorless base usually found in photographic films.

An adhesive or bonding layer is present on both sides of the base to grip the emulsion. The emulsion is but 0.01mm thick, optically clear and is the "performance" layer of the film. A final coating — called the "T coat" or "supercoat" — overlies the emulsion; its slick gelatinous nature protects the film while assisting in handling capabilities.

Suspended within the emulsion are silver-halide crystals, the light sensitive material responsible for the formation of an image. Because pure silver bromide is photographically inert, a silver bromideiodide crystal is used; the silver bromide comprises from 90 to 99 percent of the active constituents while silver iodide makes up the remaining 1 to 10 percent of the crystalline structure.

Double-coated x-ray films are rated much faster than common photographic films. Some varieties of radiographic film would be rated at a speed of 1200 ASA if this system of grading was applied within the x-ray world. Double-coated films have an image in each layer of emulsion, separated by the film base. The *parallax* phenomenon could be expected to occur in such circumstances; nevertheless, it does not ensue because the layers of emulsion are so close together.

CROSS-SECTION OF X-RAY FILM

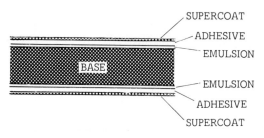

SUPERCOAT
ADHESIVE
EMULSION

BASE

EMULSION
ADHESIVE
SUPERCOAT

Fig. 5-1 — The composition of typical radiographic film.

During exposure to ionizing radiation or visible light a latent image is formed upon the film. The development process renders the latent image visible. Briefly, due to a chemical reaction during the exposure silver-sulphide atoms are formed and they become "sensitivity specks" within the crystalline structure. Silver ions are attracted to the sensitivity specks where they become converted to metallic silver during development. The metallic silver is black in color and its deposition allows for the formation of a visible image. Areas of the film receiving no radiation do not go through the silver transformation stage and consequently these areas remain light transparent.

A film that has large grains of silver halide is more sensitive to ionizing radiation or to visible light, and is known as a fast or high-speed film. Smaller crystals are present in fine-grain films, yielding better detail which requires greater exposure to produce the same degree of film blackening as a fast film.

In comparing fast and par speed films there is but one advantage to the former, that being the lessened radiation required to produce a specific film result. Par speed films offer the following advantages:

(1) They have greater margin of error;
(2) less film-crystal blurring results;
(3) they are less sensitive to scatter radiation;
(4) better film resolution occurs.

Fast films should be used only in the undesirable circumstances that an underpowered machine is being employed or an excessively large object is to be visualized; nonetheless, an inferior quality film results in comparison to the product obtainable with par speed film. Par speed films allow for the observation of fine bone detail and are a necessary requirement for quality spinographs at today's level of film manufacturing technology.

Density & Contrast

A film may be said to have good, or wide, latitude. R. J. Schulz succinctly defines this quality by stating that "latitude is used to describe the range of x-ray exposures that will produce useful photographic densities." Contrast and latitude are inversely proportional traits, i.e., increasing one automatically decreases the other. A film manufactured to be of high contrast will be of narrow latitude, and a low contrast film will have a relatively wider latitude. Exposure latitude refers to the degree of inaccuracy in the exposure time, the kilovoltage and the milliamperage which will still result in the forging of an adequate diagnostic quality picture.

Density and contrast are terms widely used in the radiographic world. Simply stated, density refers to the amount of blackness in a finished film. As greater quantities of silver are deposited on the film, it assumes a greater degree of "blackness." Because films are viewed through an illuminator this degree of blackness can be measured with an instrument called a *densitometer*. The optical density of a film can be plotted on a graph which is called the *characteristic curve* or the *H and D curve* (from "Hurter & Driffield" — the researchers who first studied characteristic curves and their relationship to light in general photography, in 1890). *Sensitometry* is the science of measuring optical densities.

From sensitometry we learn that measurement of density is done on a logarithmic basis. For example, if the metallic silver deposited upon a film allows 10 percent of the transmitted light to pass through the film, a 10:1 ratio results. The logarithm of 10 is 1 and therefore the density of this film is said to be 1. If 1 percent of the light was transmitted through the film a 100:1 ratio would result. With the log of 100 being 2, the density of this film would be 2. If only 1/1,000th of the illuminated light was to pass through the film a density of 3 would be recorded and this film would be quite black to the observer. Conversely, if 100 percent of the transmitted light passed through the film a density of zero would be recorded and this film would be completely clear.

H and D curve — or characteristic curve — valuations are important in roentgenography for the establishment of comparative film speeds, in determining exposures and in defining limits of latitude.

For the everyday x-ray user density of film is a necessary practical consideration. Milliampere-seconds directly affects film density; the greater the mAs the greater the film blackness, the lesser the mAs the lesser the film blackness. Other factors also play a subordinate although influential role. Processing methods; the density, composition and thickness of the part to be examined; film and intensifying screen combination; kilovoltage; focus-film distance —all are variable factors in the ultimate density of any roentgeno-

gram. A properly processed film comprises densities which generally vary from 0.25 in the light areas to more than 3.0 in the darkest portions.

Contrast is the visible difference between densities manifest in the completed radiograph. The final, overall level of contrast is a product of two individual components:

(1) Film contrast: that contrast which is inherent in the film. It is influenced by processing procedures and is sensitometrically plotted by the slope of the characteristic curve of a film.

(2) Subject contrast: differing anatomical structures and areas have differing beam absorption properties.

Of course, this discussion of film and subject contrast assumes the presence of ideal conditions. Scatter radiation producing fog patently reduces contrast.

Underexposure or overexposure of a film obliterates contrast. If we accept the role of contrast as improving the visibility of detail, then we must accept the corollary that a correct exposure must be made in order to obtain optimal contrast. Before a latent image can be produced upon the film, the part being examined must be adequately penetrated. The controlling factor in obtaining adequate penetration is kilovoltage.

Increasing kilovoltage increases penetration and acts to produce a long scale of contrast. Of course, if an exceedingly high kilovoltage technique is employed, the resulting film will be flat, predominantly grey and lacking in contrast. In general, a long scale of contrast is desirable, as evidenced by the illustration in Fig. 1-4. Step wedge tests reveal that 100 kVp produces low contrast — or long scale of contrast — as compared to 40 kVp. The short scale of contrast seen in high contrast films exhibits an abrupt conversion from white to black tones.

A short review of *coefficient of attenuation* is appropriate at this time. A sheet of plywood absorbs far less radiation than an equally thick sheet of aluminum, and both absorb only a fraction of an equally thick sheet of lead. Each substance absorbs, or attenuates, a definite amount of radiation. So it is with the human body. Bone absorbs more radiation than does muscle; muscle absorbs more radiation than does fat. The degree of absorption of ionizing-radiation as it passes through a particular object can be expressed by a formula which is designated as the attenuation coefficient. At higher kilovoltage levels the attenuation of radiation for bone and muscle is different than at lower kilovoltages.

Specifically, at 50 to 125 kVp and more, the density of bone has a reduced coefficient of attenuation when compared to that of soft tissues (fat, muscle). In other words, the contrast evident in bone becomes relatively less than that of soft tissues at higher kilovoltage levels. Practical use of this fact is taken advantage of in radiography of the lungs where high kVp renders the ribs ill-defined while the lung structure possesses sufficient contrast to remain diagnostically discernible.

Insofar as roentgenograms of the vertebral column's osseous structures are concerned, F. G. Bauer has conducted experiments involving thousands of films. Utilizing optimal grid and secondary scatter radiation control measures in conjunction with density equalizing filtration, it has been ascertained that the most satisfactory results are obtained with the use of 100 kVp. Films retain satisfactory contrast and the patient receives significantly lowered radiation doses than through techniques of lessened kilovoltage.

Film Fog

The greatest enemy of x-ray films is *fog*. Fog from all sources exerts an inimical effect upon all films. Fog may be defined as an undesirable darkening of film which increases its overall optical density and reduces its contrast. It is impossible to attain the total absence of fog because it is present on films even before they reach the hands of the x-ray user. The *base fog* is always present and can be measured with a densitometer. Reduced to its lowest common denominator, base fog is simply base-plus-fog. The film base is either a clear base or, most commonly, a blue base, the latter having a minimal amount of blue pigment included by the manufacturer. If a particular film is fixed without being exposed to ionizing radiation, or subjected to the development process, a densitometer reading in the order of 0.05 to 0.07 usually is recorded. This is the *inherent optical density* or base density of a film.

Next, an unexposed film is subjected to the normal processing steps of development, rinse, fixation and final rinse previous to appraisal with a densitometer. The result is the amount of base fog present in the film before it is subjected to ionizing radiation. The former measurement for base density can be subtracted from this figure, revealing the extent of fog density present. An acceptable level of base fog is 0.2 or less. The authors have conducted tests where films direct from the distributor contained base fog levels of 0.25, 0.27, 0.30 and even higher. Such films have an inbuilt greyness, precluding satisfactory diagnostic results irrespective of the attention paid to all other roentgenographic details.

On rare occasions a manufacturer inadvertently will allow faulty film to leave the factory. Films may be stored too long by the manufacturer or the distributor. From production point in the factory to delivery to the user, film storage and transport are of critical significance. Users should always ensure that they receive fresh film and that they put it into service before its expiry date. Films may be stored at too high a temperature, or in an area of high humidity. Films may be subject to cosmic radiation, ionizing radiation or harmful chemical fumes before delivery to the consumer. All of the foregoing increase the base fog level of film and reduce the diagnostic capabilities of those examinations using the pre-fogged material. Obviously, no manufacturer wants to supply purchasers with inferior quality materials. Nevertheless, base fog levels do differ significantly between various makers and it behooves the aware consumer to be informed of the best quality film available in his/her locale.

Remember that fast films are more sensitive than par speed films and that they will fog quicker than their slower counterparts. We will return to the topic of fog soon, during discussion of film protection, and again in Chapter IX when considering the darkroom. Fog is certainly the arch foe of quality roentgenographic work; every day it mars diagnostic excellence — most usually unnecessarily.

Quantum Mottle

Theory holds that radiation is apportioned and transmitted through space in discrete quanta, or separate bundles, rather than in a continuous, evenly balanced manner. The effect that these separate bundles of x-rays have upon films is known as *quantum mottle*. Visibly, quantum mottle is revealed as a "spotty" or grainy appearance upon the film.

The simplest analogy to illustrate quantum mottle is the one put forth by the Kodak Company in a trade publication several years ago. If rain falls heavily upon a section of sidewalk the entire area will be wetted evenly, if not in actual fact at least in appearance. If however, rain falls lightly upon an equivalent area of sidewalk the degree of wetting will be irregular and uneven, both in actual fact and in appearance. Differences in rainfall are quite noticeable with a light fall and imperceptible with a heavy shower. So it is with x-ray. The use of very high speed screens can reduce the required exposure to such a degree that the film does not receive an overall, even dose of radiation

before density requisites are met. Thus there is a granular or spotty appearance to the final film product.

Quantum mottle is a comparatively recent encumbrance to modern radiography, since the advent of extremely fast films and screens. Films taken of, for example, the cervical area via par speed screens and par speed films will not be subject to quantum mottle. Films taken in the lumbar area would be affected by quantum mottle if exposures were attempted with fast film and super-fast rare earth screens. You may see the term *noise* used to describe either mottle or artifacts found on the x-ray film.

Detail

Various writers look at film detail from different viewpoints. One proclaims detail to be composed of sharpness and visibility. A second states that detail is sharpness and contrast. A third asserts it to be contrast and definition. Yet another declares that all films have detail and the sharpness of the recorded image is the definition.

By the detractive method let us look at what causes *unsharpness* in films. Movement unsharpness results when the tube, film or part being examined is set in motion during the exposure. A large focal spot will yield geometric unsharpness; so will a short focus-film distance or a long object-film distance. Very fast intensifying screens yield inherent unsharpness. Poor contact between screen and film produces further unsharpness. This perceived unsharpness results in loss of detail to the film and a consequent reduction in diagnostic value. What can the eye see? Unsharpness is observable when two reference points are 0.2mm apart; standard viewbox illumination precludes discernment at lesser intervals.

How does one obtain good definition? By reducing scatter radiation and its consequent fog; by using the smallest allowable focal spot, shortest object-film distance and longest focus-film distance practicable; by immobilizing the relevant body part; by using the most appropriate film-screen combination and making sure both components are in good contact; by controlling distortion and magnification through appropriate techniques; by eliminating patient and tube movement; in short, by paying attention to all details.

Film Care & Protection

Let us assume that a quantity of film has been delivered to your door, conveyed safely, endowed with minimal base fog and in a state of readiness for the task at hand. What measures are undertaken to insure that the film remains unsullied?

Even if an x-ray room is lead-lined all films except the one in immediate use should be stored in one of two lead boxes. (If the room is lead-lined a lead box is still essential to prevent fogging from patient/equipment sources.) It is a good idea to order the lead boxes before ordering the first box of film. One lead-lined box should be located in the darkroom, the other near the x-ray unit itself if that is where cassettes are situated during an examination. To foil the effects of stray radiation it is necessary to provide lead shielding for all films (except the one being exposed) when the x-ray machine is in use. As discussed earlier, the greatest **enemy of diagnostic radiography is fog**. Stray radiation is a peerless cause of fog which, through inattention to detail, results in the production of unacceptable radiographs by careless x-ray users.

The lead boxes should be constructed of "three pound lead," i.e., lead of 1.5mm thickness or more. All six sides of each box should be leaded and, for assured protection, the lead of the opening lid or door should overlap that of the four sides. Dividers allowing cassettes and film boxes to be "pigeonholed" should be installed; cassette surfaces are susceptible to damage if handled carelessly. Storage space should be orientated vertically;

film packets should never be stacked on top of each other where they can be subjected to undue pressure.

An interesting experiment will illustrate the degree of protection films have received. Extract a fresh film from a newly delivered box and remove another stored film, one in your possession the longest, and process both equally. Develop both films together, agitating jointly, fix and rinse identically. Now compare them in equivalent lighting. The fresh film will probably be more transparent, less grey. This will be especially noticeable if stray radiation reached the older film, producing fog. Unequivocally, fog will result if films are stored without the benefit of lead's protection. Neither is it good enough to keep unexposed films in steel boxes; they must be stored in lead-lined containers for complete protection.

Films last much longer if kept at lower temperatures, preferably below 20°C (68°F). In fact, freezing film is not harmful to the emulsion as long as the sealed package is warmed to room temperature before opening, averting moisture formation on the film.

A humidity range of 50 to 60 percent is ideal. High humidity will alter the film's speed while low humidity — below 30 percent — will increase the likelihood of static occurring.

Buying film in small lots assures freshness. A good rule is never to have more than one sealed package of film in readiness for each opened box already in use. For best results load cassettes immediately prior to their intended use; films "age" faster in cassettes. Load films on a clean work bench and maintain darkroom benches and floors in a dust-free state.

Fingernails, when pressured against film, will "fracture" the emulsion, yielding artifacts resembling half-moons or quarter-moons. Obviously, cassettes must be loaded in total darkness; any white light reaching the film will produce instant blackening.

Film is supplied with or without interleaving paper for each individual sheet. Interleaving does help to protect the film, providing a margin-of-error advantage. However, interleaved films do cost more. A somewhat surprising result of tests conducted by x-ray workers suggests that the radioactivity level in the interleaving paper may even contribute to film fogging. If films are stored directly in bins instead of within manufacturers' cartons, the film bin must be light-and radiation-proof or fogging will surely ensue.

The following list enumerates factors which conflict with the attainment of diagnostic quality radiographs. Protect films from:

> Heat
> White Light
> Safelight
> Chemicals
> Chemical Fumes - Vapors of formalin, ammonia, hydrogen sulphide, various cleaning agents and polishes will fog films.
> Compression
> Contaminated Fingers - Moist, greasy, metallic or chemically laden digits can damage film, especially before development.
> Fingernails
> Abrasions
> Lighted Cigarettes
> Static Electricity
> Background and Ionizing Radiation

Static Electricity

Static electricity may discharge onto nonprocessed x-ray film, creating a diverse array of artifacts. K. Jackson places static varieties into one of three groups:

(1) Tree Static
(2) Crown Static
(3) Smudge Static

Tree static bears a resemblance to its namesake and is believed to originate from rapid film movements; e.g., hurried withdrawal of film from package or bin. It is particularly noticeable when a sheet of interleaving paper is hastily drawn away from the film. Crown static usually manifests itself near the film border, often appearing following rapid film withdrawal from a tightly packed box. Smudge static tends to occur over a relatively large area of film, the discharge following a route ordained by dust or dirt particles on damaged screen surfaces.

Static most often is noticed during periods of low atmospheric humidity. According to Jackson the ability of moisture in the air around the film to promote the dissipation of excessive static charges is the greatest aid in the prevention of static. Bench tops, type of clothing worn, carpeting and even cassettes can all be sources of static electricity.

How is static minimized? By careful film handling; by maintaining proper storage temperature and humidity conditions; by avoiding orlon or nylon garments and rubber-soled shoes; by allowing for earthing in the darkroom where conductive floors are made of concrete, terrazzo or conductive rubber (rubber mats, cork or linoleum floors to be avoided); and by ensuring darkroom cleanliness, including prudent screen care.

<u>Practical Perspective</u>

<u>SCATTER RADIATION</u>

THIS FILM WAS EXPOSED BY BACKSCATTER RADIATION AT A DISTANCE OF 10 FEET FROM THE PATIENT

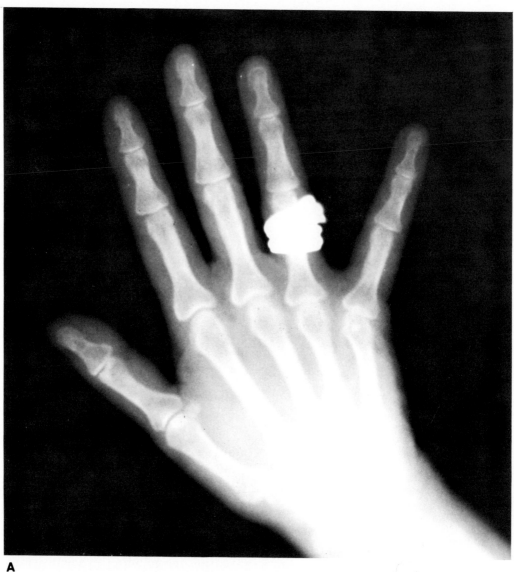

A

THIS FILM WAS EXPOSED
BY BACKSCATTER RADIATION
AT A DISTANCE OF 10 FEET
FROM THE PATIENT

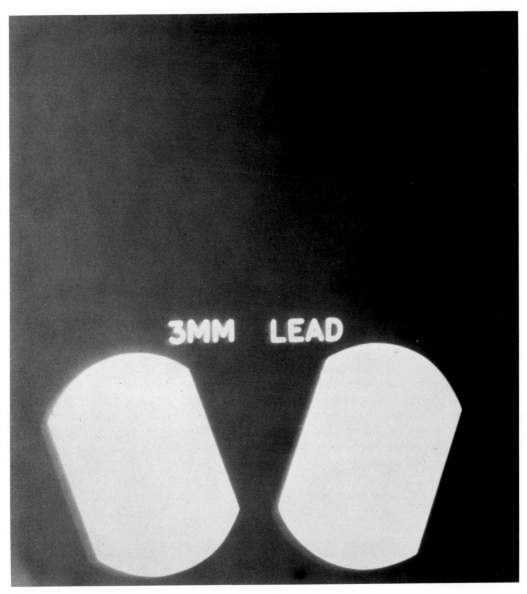

B

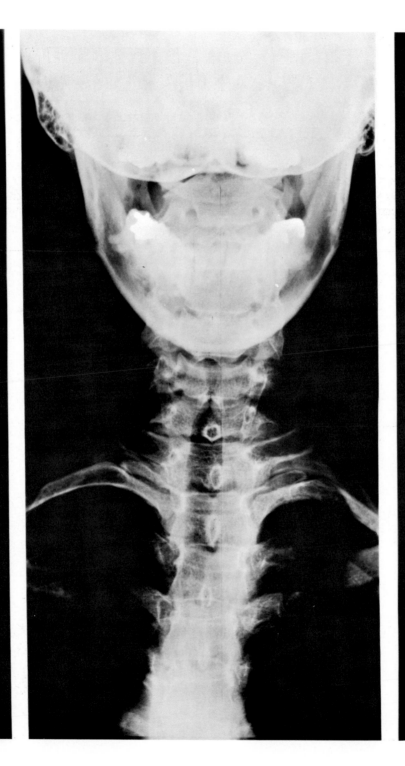

RIGHT SIDE

MRS E M RUSSEL

STANDING POSITION

21 JUNE

F.G. BAUER
CHIROPRACTOR

c

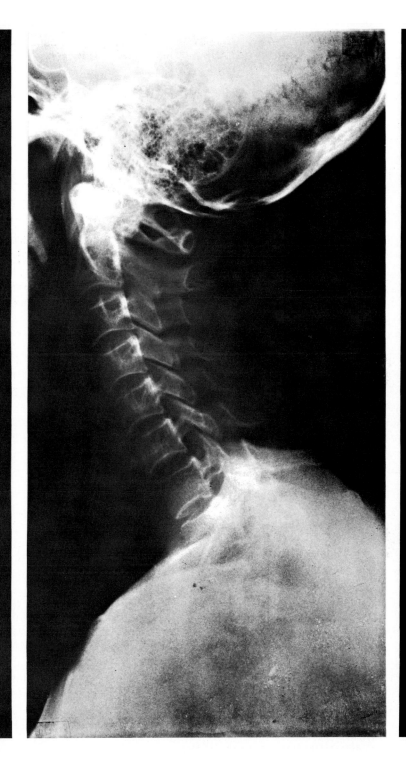

STANDING POSITION

21 JUNE

F.G. BAUER
CHIROPRACTOR

RIGHT SIDE

MRS E M RUSSEL

D

In varying degrees, scatter radiation encumbers all x-ray films. Scatter contributes to final film density but not in a positive manner; rather, increased scatter leads to lessened contrast and generalized image degradation. The radiograph suffering from excessive scatter radiation appears to be grey overall, as dull and flat as snow at winter's end.

Determinants of scatter include the thickness and density of the part being examined, the field size and the kVp being employed. The x-ray user can do nothing about the density of the anatomical part. In some instances compression helps by reducing tissue thickness. Tight collimation reduces scatter; it is always a recommended procedure. Filtration reduces scatter. To a degree filtration attenuates all radiation. However, longer wavelength, lower kilovoltage radiation is diminished more than shorter wavelength, higher kilovoltage radiation. In toto, reducing radiation decreases scatter radiation. Low kVp decreases scatter. Unfortunately, low kVp may produce unsatisfactory radiographic penetration and it definitely produces elevated patient exposure values. The high/optimal (100) kVp technique advocated in this text increases the scatter yield in comparison to 70-80 kVp techniques. That is why a quality grid must be used to clean-up scatter radiation. Many x-ray users are unaware of the ease with which films become "fogged" from scatter radiation. The x-ray films reproduced in this section were chosen to illustrate the effects of scatter in normal radiographic working conditions.

The "scatter hand" demonstrated herein stands out clearly, considering the circumstances of the exposure. A cassette loaded with Siemens Special intensifying screens and Agfa RPl film was placed on the wall opposite to a simulated patient being examined in front of a wall bucky. A plastic bucket filled with water was used to simulate the human body. The beam was collimated to 10″ x 12″ (25cm x 30cm) and the FFD was 48″ (122cm). The factors for the exposure were 100 kVp and 500 mAs. The test film placed against the wall was 10′ (305cm) from the patient, almost in line with direct backscatter, or nearly 180° away from the alignment of the central ray.

The test subject placed her hand upon the cassette and the x-ray machine was activated. The initial experiment was done at 100 kVp and 100 mAs. The image from this exposure was quite visible but it lacked resolution. This is understandable when one recalls that scatter radiation comes from all directions, not from a small focal spot. The film resulting from the 100 kVp-500 mAs test is reproduced in Fig. (A). As can be seen, osseous bone detail is remarkably distinct.

Fig. (B) is a similar test involving the application of gonadal shields of 3mm lead thickness to the front of the test cassette. Factors again used were 100 kVp and 500 mAs but this time the FFD was increased to 80″ (200cm). Although radiation had to travel significantly further to reach the test film, the image in Fig. (B) is quite well defined. If the clarity of illustrations (A) and (B) have surprised you somewhat, the tests have been a success. X-ray users sometimes forget just how harmful scatter radiation can be to radiographic quality.

The two cervical radiographs shown in Fig. (C) and (D) provide a good comparison of the inimical effects of scatter radiation. The lateral cervical film was taken in the usual manner but it was then inadvertently left resting midway between the focal spot and the patient, and approximately 5′ (150cm) lateral to the central ray. The A-P view was then taken, with exposure factors of 100 kVp and 50 mAs. Detail screens were used in combination with Dupont 2 DC film in both exposures. The overall grey appearance of the lateral cervical film is due to the effects of scatter radiation from just one exposure.

All films except the one being used must be kept protected within lead-lined containers to assure protection against scatter radiation.

Chapter **6**

Screens & Cassettes

Diagnostic x-rays in the U.S. without doubt result in the saving of hundreds of thousands of lives each year, but this is no excuse for using them carelessly and excessively so as to cause the needless loss of tens of thousands of lives each year.

K. Z. Morgan, *Reducing Medical Exposure to Ionizing Radiation*, 36:358-68, p. 366, American Industrial Hygiene Association Journal, 1975.

Intensifying Screens

Modern technology is bringing about evolutionary changes in radiographic screens, changes that could be described as near revolutionary in development. After many years of seemingly static conditions the nineteen-sixties and seventies have witnessed rapid proliferation of faster and faster intensifying screens. Our purpose in this chapter is to enhance understanding for the x-ray user, remain practical in orientation while at the same time touching upon developments that will undoubtedly alter radiographic methods considerably in the years ahead.

X-ray film has a relatively low sensitivity to ionizing radiation. This poses no problems in exposing a hand or a toe whereby a satisfactory image can be made without the aid of screens, i.e., with non-screen film. However, in order to view the vertebral column or pelvis without the benefit of intensifying screens, the exposure required is so great that the x-ray dose issued to the patient would prohibit the examination from taking place. As an example, a lateral lumbar exposure undertaken with the aid of high speed intensifying screens which would yield an optimal result with the use of 100 kVp and 250 mAs would, without screens, require factors of 100 kVp and 19,900 mAs!

Intensifying screens are so-called because their function is to multiply or intensify the photographic effect of ionizing radiation. Conventional films do not respond well to direct x-ray exposure. An intermediary substance is required to multiply the photographic effect just mentioned, and to lessen the radiation dose received by the patient. Intensifying screens are the agents performing this essential function. They exhibit the property of fluorescence which means that upon excitation visible light is emitted. Ionizing radiation reaches the screen's active layer, containing crystals — collectively called phosphors — and the crystals convert the x-ray energy into

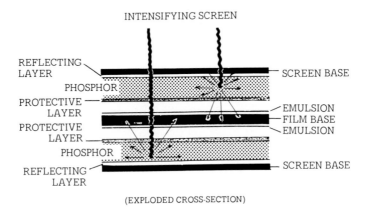

INTENSIFYING SCREEN

REFLECTING
LAYER
PHOSPHOR
PROTECTIVE
LAYER
PROTECTIVE
LAYER
PHOSPHOR
REFLECTING
LAYER

SCREEN BASE
EMULSION
FILM BASE
EMULSION
SCREEN BASE

(EXPLODED CROSS-SECTION)

Fig. 6-1 — Relationship of intensifying screens to film within cassette. The photographic effect of x-ray photons is multiplied by the phosphor of the intensifying screens.

light energy which causes the formation of a latent image on the film.

Conventional screens emit light in the blue-violet range of the spectrum, which is that portion of the spectrum producing the greatest photographic effect. Each x-ray photon reaching a medium speed screen results in the creation of approximately 1,000 light photons. The human eye is not especially sensitive to blue-violet wave-lengths and it perceives, or "sees," luminous screens as violet in color when they are fluorescing.

The use of intensifying screens is almost as old as the discovery of x-ray. More than 80 years ago pioneering x-ray workers used calcium tungstate crystals as the phosphor of choice for intensifying screens and today this compound remains the first choice in a large variety of screen applications. Calcium tungstate ($CaWO^4$) is predictable, reliable, physically sturdy, reacts generally in a linear manner to kilovoltage changes and has a relatively high coefficiency of x-ray absorption. Simply stated, x-ray photons strike the calcium tungstate crystals within the screen, causing the crystals to fluoresce. Thus the original x-ray energy is transformed into visible light which greatly magnifies the effect of the original exposure. Remember that x-ray radiation does not have a particularly vigorous

photographic effect and in a comparative sense, radiographic film is much more sensitive to the rays of visible light.

The cross-sectioned view of a representative screen comprises four layers, as illustrated in Fig. 6-1. The base is made of plastic upon which a reflecting layer is applied. This layer is commonly titanium oxide, a reflecting medium which directs visible light towards the film. The active stratum is the phosphor layer, containing calcium tungstate for example, suspended in a clear matrix. Coating the phosphor is a plastic protective layer which provides physical protection for the phosphor, allows the screen to be cleaned and helps to prevent static formation.

The speed of intensifying screens depends upon two factors:

1. The thickness of the phosphor layer of the screen, and
2. The size of the phosphor's crystals.

Generally speaking, the thicker the phosphor layer in a screen, the faster the screen speed will be. Greater fluorescence results from thicker screens, causing greater conversion of x-ray energy to visible light energy. Of course, greater thickness causes greater diffusion of light with its attendant loss of resolution. Some manufacturers include varying amounts of dye in their screens. The dye

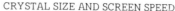

CRYSTAL SIZE AND SCREEN SPEED

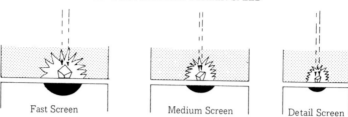

Fast Screen   Medium Screen   Detail Screen

Fig. 6-2 — Increased size of screen crystals increases the speed and decreases the definition of intensifying screens.

assists in curtailing light diffusion, thereby giving the screens better resolution.

(At this time it is appropriate to recall that "everything in x-ray is a compromise." The best detail can be obtained without screens but the dosage engendered is prohibitive. Fast films reduce patient dosage but the loss of bone detail may cause an early pathology to be missed. The radiographic answer is almost invariably a compromise, one that strives for greatest clarity with the least amount of radiation issued for existing circumstances.)

As referred to in Fig. 6-2, large crystals increase the screen's speed, often in a ratio of direct proportions. As the crystals diminish in size the resolution improves. In actuality screen grain size is not comparable to film grain size. The diameter of a silver halide crystal is approximately one micron, while the diameter of screen phosphors is from five to ten microns or more. This explains why screen-films can never hope to compete with non-screen-films for detail. Technological advances in screens have benefitted x-ray users and patients — the latter via reduced radiation dosages, the former via improved diagnostic capabilities. Today's very fast screens cause no more kinetic blurring than par speed screens once did.

In addition to the customary thickness/size considerations for determining screen speed, increasing kVp will augment screen speed. Higher kVp produces higher

energy; the higher energy radiation striking the phosphor causes more light to emanate from the crystals, thereby effectively increasing the screen's speed.

The amount of "work" accomplished by intensifying screens is quite miraculous. Mr. Ken Jackson, technical specialist with the Dupont organization, kindly provided the figures that are used in the chart set out in Fig. 6-3. As illustrated, a non-screen x-ray film achieves its final density without benefit of any screen intensification at all. The work performed by average high definition (or fine detail) screens equals 95 percent while that done by the film comprises just 5 percent of the final density. In the case of today's rare earth screens the film is responsible for 0.5 percent of blackening, the intensifying screens providing the remaining 99.5 percent of film density. It can be readily appreciated that intensifying screens are well worth looking after.

A similar depiction, in this instance expressing exposure times based on par speed screens representing a one second exposure, is shown in Fig. 6-4.

Screen speeds continue to increase and there is reason to anticipate further refinement in years ahead. What about the best combination of film and screen for today's vertebral imaging requirements? Par-speed films and high speed screens produce the optimal result. Extremely sensitive, or high speed films are not recommended; they are more susceptible to the effects of heat, compression, stray

Fig. 6-3

Percentage of Work Done by Screens	%
1. X-ray film	0
2. Non-screen film	0
3. Dental film	0
4. Dupont detail screens	90
5. Average high definition screens	95
6. Par speed screens	97.5
7. High speed screens	98.75
8. Extra high-speed screens	99
9. Dupont Lightning Plus screens	99.17
10. Rare earth or equivalent screens	99.5
11. Quanta III screens	99.7

Fig. 6-4

Relative Exposure Times	Seconds
1. Non-screen film	40
2. Detail screens	4
3. Fast detail screens	2
4. Par-speed screens	1
5. High speed screens	0.5
6. High plus screens	0.4
7. Lightning plus screens	0.32
8. Quanta II screens	0.2
9. Quanta III screens	0.12

radiation, etc., and they normally have a shorter shelf life. The compromise in radiographic variables mandates very fast screens and par speed film for thicker body parts. For comparatively thinner areas — i.e., the cervical spine — high definition screens remain acceptable. Radiation quantities are not so prodigious when dealing with the cervical region and slower screens do yield excellent detail in this area of tight collimation opportunities.

Screen speeds for identical descriptive labels vary considerably among manufacturers, so much so that a label of, for example, high definition is no more than a guide to the relative speed of a particular screen. Film speeds are also demonstrably different among brands purporting to be graded at parity. This entire situation has been confusing for many years and the only sure way of ascertaining film-screen speeds in combination is by experimentation.

Rare Earth Intensifying Screens

The term "rare earth" refers to a group of phosphors which have been developed into commercial availability during the past decade. The label came about to indicate the effort needed to prepare these elements for radiographic usage; rare earth elements are not truly uncommon or scarce. The difficulties in processing are reflected in the cost of these screens which often are twice as expensive as calcium tungstate screens.

It is the qualities possessed by rare earth screens that have made them exciting, qualities that portend well for continuing advances in the technology of screen phosphors. The two ultimate objectives in screen function are speed and resolution. Rare earth screens have the potential to approach these dual goals. There is an increased conversion efficiency with rare earth phosphors, i.e., rare earth screens are more effective in converting radiant energy into the energy of visible light. The conversion efficiency of calcium tungstate screens is approximately 5 percent while that of rare earth screens varies from 13 to 20 percent.

There are many factors pointing towards the increased employment of rare earth phosphors. In some instances the use of rare earth screens can obviate the need for more powerful generators; certainly the efficiency of low-powered equipment is increased. The operational life of tubes may be able to be extended through the use of rare earth phosphors. Coatings of these screens are generally thinner, allowing increased screen-film contact. Reduction in screen thickness points towards improved film resolution. Some manufacturers claim that there is a decreased sensitivity to scatter radiation ("scatter rejection") and a consequent improvement in contrast levels through the use of rare earth materials. Further, it is claimed that the silver content of a film used in conjunction with rare earth screens can be of a lessened magnitude. If this assertion proves to be correct it will be a real boon to x-ray users. Silver content in films is dropping already and the volatile tendencies of world metal markets gives scant encouragement to the hope for a return to "normal" film silver levels.

The new screens possess an efficiency twice that of calcium tungstate screens. Stated another way it means that exposures can be cut in half without experiencing a penalty. This then is the ultimate fascination of the new technology, that it may be possible to maintain film quality while reducing the radiation dose to the patient by 50 percent or more.

After painting a readers' rainbow it must be said that the pot of gold is not at the rainbow's end, at least not yet. There are still hitches in the utilization of rare earth phosphors. Image noise — which will be discussed shortly — increases with rare earth screens. The rapidly reacting phosphors are so fast that the margin for error in radiographic techniques is correspondingly diminshed. Some very effective phosphors have been found but they are so hydroscopic that they cannot be used in intensifying screens. Such is the case with cesium iodide, utilized in image intensifiers. A drop of 15 to 25 percent in the speed of rare earth screens has been noted within a period of twelve months. It is claimed that the phosphors are now "stabilized" to prevent this rapid downgrading from occurring.

The wavelength of a phosphor must be appropriate before it can be used for radiographic purposes. Calcium tungstate emits in the blue-violet to ultraviolet portion of the spectrum. Barium fluorochloride and lanthanum oxybromide phosphors also are situated in the blue-light spectrum while gadolinium oxysulfide and lanthanum oxysulfide emit light mainly in the green area of the visible spectrum. This means that a special film and a specific safelight must be used with green-emitting phosphors.

Noise

Noise refers to the blotchy, mottled appearance of an x-ray film. Noise can result from the random statistical fluctuations in the distribution of photons upon the film's surface. This is true quantum mottle. Attempting to produce a diagnostic film with a comparatively small number of x-ray photons leads to the appearance of quantum mottle. Rare earth screens absorb more x-ray energy and convert more of this absorbed energy into visible light. Consequently, there is a greater tendency for quantum mottle to appear during the use of rare earth screens than during the use of calcium tungstate screens. It can be said that in general an increase in quantum mottle — noise — accompanies an increase in the speed of a screen-film combination.

Screen noise may be termed screen grain or screen structure mottle. It results from inconsistencies in the manufacturing process which allow crystals to clump together in a less than homogenous fashion. It is not common and should be entirely absent from well-produced intensifying screens.

Care of Intensifying Screens

Because atoms in the phosphor regroup themselves to their initial positions after an x-ray exposure, screens should maintain their efficiency for several years, and many do. With proper care screens will give years of reliable service; with improper care they may be worthless within a few months. Rough handling, incorrect insertion and removal of films and unsound cleaning methods are all factors leading to the early demise of intensifying screens. Well cared-for screens, used with circumspection, should last in the neighborhood of ten years. Just to be prudent, remember how little they cost you initially, how well they served you over the years, and then retire screens after seven years' duty.

Intensifying screens require regular care in order to continue performing efficaciously. An "information slip" is provided by most manufacturers, furnishing instructions for maintaining screen efficiency. A good location for affixing this leaflet is the darkroom wall, where it is available for ready reference. For example, some screens can be cleaned with mild soap and water, some with anti-static preparations, and others only with ethyl alcohol. Individual manufacturers supply directions for their respective products. When cleaning screens remember not to use an excessive amount of liquid cleaning agent. An imperfect edge seal will allow moisture to enter, leading to the ultimate destruction of the intensifying screens.

New screens must be installed in a cassette of sound condition, if not in a new cassette. Examine the cassette face with particular attention to ensure that no indentations are present. Screen contact may be lost in an irregular-surfaced cassette and this combination will forevermore yield one or more areas suffering from loss of detail.

In the past screens were affixed within cassettes by a type of glue that occasionally allowed the glue to work its way upwards to the front of the screen. This does not happen with the "ripple tape" material which is currently used as an adhesive in modern screens. This tape may be flat or slightly corrugated. In either instance make sure that the cassette is clean before installing the screen. Once the screen is centered within the cassette— there may be enough edge space to allow a degree of offcentering — close the cassette with a double thickness of interleaving paper separating the screen surfaces. Leave the cassette closed overnight and by morning a permanently and securely affixed pair of screens will be ready for use. Do not use additional adhesive beyond that found on the screen tape.

Screens labelled "FRONT" or "FORDER-FOLIE" (German) should be mounted within the tube side of the cassette. Screens labelled "BACK" or "RUECK-FOLIE" (German) are then mounted on the opposing cassette surface.

The back screen was thicker than the front screen in early model screen pairs. This thicker layer of phosphor trapped more x-ray photons and, from a practical standpoint, necessitated care in installing the correct screen in the correct location. To this day many screens maintain a thickness differential. However, other screen pairs are of equal thickness and with these models it matters not which screen is applied to the front or the back of a cassette.

A clean, dust-free darkroom will help to keep foreign objects out of screens. Even such a simple thing as the mundane act of sneezing near an open cassette could cause severe screen damage. A bright incandescent light in the darkroom allows for a thorough inspection to be made of screens. An appropriate vacuum cleaner attachment is very helpful in keeping potential artifacts away from the screen surface; a periodic vacuuming is recommended for thorough screen care.

Careless extraction of a film from the cassette could prove destructive to the intensifying screens. Should a film steadfastly adhere to a screen by atmospheric pressure, the attempted removal by "digging" the film away from the screen with a fingernail is an open invitation to permanent screen damage.

It is a good idea to perform a brief screen check on a daily basis. Certainly, if an artifact is noticed on a processed radiograph the foreign object should be removed immediately from the relevant screen. A safe way to wipe a screen is with a piece of household facial tissue. If this is inadequate to dislodge the foreign object a soft wooden match generally suffices; scrape against the artifact with light pressure to avoid damaging the screen.

Cassettes

Cassette functions are significant and simple: to furnish light-free environment for the film and to provide for faultless film-screen contact.

As previously discussed, rough handl-

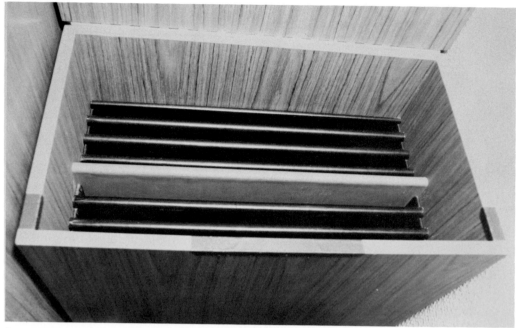

A   **PROPER**

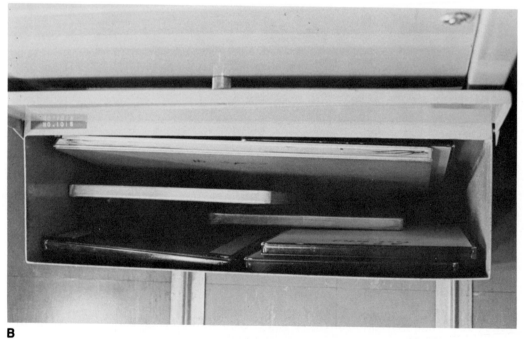

B

IMPROPER

Fig. 6-5 — "A" & "B" proper and improper methods of cassette storage in an x-ray room.

ing soon engenders regional areas of poor film-screen contact and may even induce light leaks. A simple experiment allows one to check the light-proof status of a cassette. Load the cassette with a sheet of fresh film, expose it with the back side to intense white light for a few moments and then develop the film in the usual way. If portions of the film are fogged, or there are grey-black streaks on the film, light has found a way to enter the cassette.

Cassettes are designed to provide absolute film-screen contact. Anything less allows image unsharpness to occur wherever light rays are permitted to disperse. The best quality high definition screens may not produce as sharp a film result as ultra high speed screens if film-screen contact is lost or unevenly distributed.

When ordering cassettes make sure that lead-backed models are specified. The lead lining is necessary to prevent radiation from re-entering the cassette and fogging the film. Using a marking pen or pencil, identify all cassettes to indicate which end is superior. There is never a doubt as to the upper end during any exposure if this is done, and it facilitates the loading of films into hangers "topside up," the logical way to develop radiographs.

Numerous measures can be undertaken to further cassette longevity. Cassettes should be stored upright, the vertical position helping to maintain cassette integrity. Padded, individual, vertically-oriented slots or compartments are the safest form of cassette storage. Do not carry two or more cassettes together without adequate padding between them. Try to avoid carrying two cassettes of unequal size together. Likewise, use all care to avoid dropping cassettes or knocking them against each other, or striking surrounding objects. Wherever possible use one kind of cassette, which aids in reducing possible darkroom confusion. Fig. 6-5 demonstrates one reason why some cassettes last for years while others have a lifespan of only months.

Practical Perspective

TESTING SCREEN CONTACT

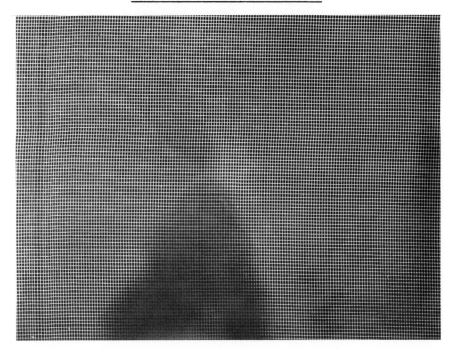

One of the most readily feasible ways of testing for intensifying screen contact is by the well-known wire screen procedure. A piece of fine wire mesh is placed in close contact with the front of a loaded cassette. The most suitable and easily obtainable material is copper screening; aluminum or plastic screening is too light to be an efficient absorber of x-rays. The wire can be taped to the cassette without damaging the cassette in any way.

This combination is then exposed and processed. Good screen contact will result in a sharp image of the wire and even density across the entire film. Poor screen contact will reveal indistinct, blurred wire screening and increased density in the area/s of faulty contact. Because of the difficulty in maintaining even pressure over larger areas, this problem is more likely to arise in 14" x 17" cassettes than, for example, in 8" x 10" cassettes.

Unless the fault is a minor one any cassette found to be defective should be discarded. All cassettes are subject to wear and tear and even the best must be replaced periodically.

Chapter 7

A. — Collimation

B. — Filtration

Whatever the type of exposure, it is always important to restrict the radiation to the smallest possible area in order to reduce the radiation hazard to the patient and to improve contrast.

G. J. Van Deer Plaats, *Medical X-Ray Technique*, p. 311, Philips Technical Library, 1969.

Filters are simple and inexpensive. Nowhere else in radiology do we gain so much for so little money.

E. E. Christensen, T. S. Curry, J. E. Dowdey, *An Introduction to the Physics of Diagnostic Radiology*, p. 82, 2nd Edition, Lea & Febiger, 1978.

Collimation

One of the most effective methods of minimizing patient radiation exposure is by the use of a collimator, or light-beam diaphragm (LBD) as it is called in some countries. Proper use of a collimator ensures that the smallest possible field is irradiated, consequently lessening the volume of tissue exposed.

Not all that many years ago the cone and slot diaphragm were the mainstays of beam restriction devices. Neither performed particularly well but they did exercise a degree of control over the area to be exposed, and the cone offered visual assistance in directing the central ray to the center of the film. The advent of collimators brought about the first genuinely competent means of limiting the field of view for each and every exposure.

The collimator is so efficacious that various governmental agencies have mandated its use. In the United States, for example, all new x-ray installations must be fitted with automatic collimation apparatus, termed "positive beam limitation." Such a device will prevent an exposure from occurring unless the beam is collimated to match the size of the cassette being used.

How does a collimator function? The illustration in Fig. 7-1 demonstrates the salient features of an "LBD." The light bulb is placed to the side of the beam,

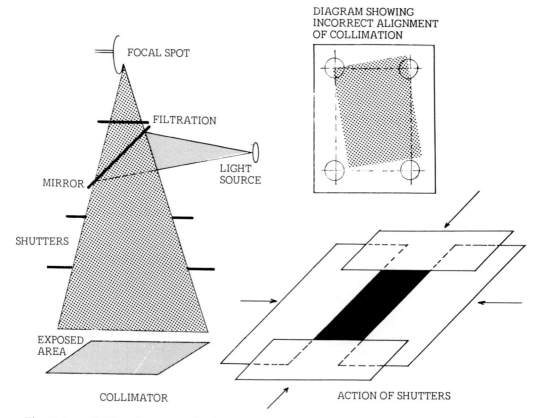

Fig. 7-1 — Collimation controls the size of the x-ray beam and the volume of tissue irradiated.

reflecting light from the mirror onto the subject of the imaging examination. The cross section of the mirrored light is controlled by the collimator's shutters. This light-beam corresponds directly in size to the cross section of the x-ray beam. The shutters are lead, each pair moving independently of the other pair, the beam modified to any number of possible configurations in the square/rectangular modes.

Remember that the collimator is often used at Focus Film Distances (FFD) of 91cm — 100cm (36" — 40"). Any error in collimation will be magnified if an FFD of greater length is utilized. Clinicians interested in biomechanical investigation often utilize a 150cm — 200cm (60" —80") FFD; collimation inaccuracies become readily discernible at these longer distances.

Collimator Alignment

Most collimator light bulbs have a limited lifespan. While it is usually a simple task to change these bulbs, a newly installed model often reveals a slight degree of misalignment. Even the filament of the bulb can be inexactly located in relation to the bayonet fitting. Thus, it is necessary to recheck alignment with the installation of each new bulb.

It is best to check collimator alignment at the usual operating distance (FFD) and, naturally, it is ordinarily easier to correct the path of the light beam than it is to alter the direction of the x-ray beam.

Begin by placing the largest size cassette used in the bucky tray; the popular 35cm x 43cm (14" x 17") size cassette will suffice. Ascertain whether a vertical mid-line would bisect the cassette as well as the bucky front. If a discrepancy exists, one of two solutions will rectify the situation.

Make an appropriate adjustment to the bucky tray arrester so that cassette and bucky midlines now coincide. If this cannot be accomplished the front surface of the bucky can be imprinted with a "new" vertical line. The line will indicate the location of the cassette center when the tray is in its normal operating position.

Obtain a superseded intensifying screen of a "fast" speed for greatest luminescence. Tape it accurately to the bucky front so that it overlies the cassette precisely. Inscribe a vertical line through the middle of the screen, ensuring that it coincides with an equivalent line in the center of the cassette.

Mark out a square on the screen, 20cm (8") in breadth, so that the vertical line bisects the square. Using the greatest FFD employed during imaging examinations turn on the collimator light and align it perfectly to this square. (It is worth noting that the shutters of the collimator often move unevenly, one side commonly lagging behind the other side upon opening. Suggested procedure calls for maximum shutter opening followed by closing of shutters until the desired border is obtained.) Apply markers within the 20cm square; they will allow for orientation of the film which will be taken shortly.

The room must be sufficiently darkened to prevent ambient light from "dimming" the collimator light source. The illuminated square should be readily distinguishable when the operator stations himself at the exposure button. Turn the collimator light off.

Make an exposure of one second's duration. Watch for the blue-purple light which appears on the intensifying screen. Develop the exposed film in the usual way. If the exposure-illuminated area corresponds exactly to the collimator-illuminated area there is no need to adjust the x-ray beam or the collimator.

If either beam or collimator are out of alignment, corrective measures must be taken. When an asymmetrical field is visible on the processed film, tube alignment must be rectified. When the collimator is improperly directed its accuracy must be reestablished. Various adjustments are possible depending, of course, upon the make and model of collimator. The bulb and/or bulb socket may be capable of adjustment. The collimator mirror often is amenable to alignment correction procedures.

It is extremely important that the field size in any imaging examination be kept at the minimum consistent with clinical objectives. Therefore, any problem or malfunctioning which occurs in the collimator that cannot be easily corrected by the x-ray user necessitates the attention of appropriate service personnel.

Radiation & Collimation

Strict use of the collimator will enhance any x-ray film. The quality of the radiograph will be improved and the patient will receive considerably less radiation. The film quality is improved because scatter radiation is decreased. It does not matter what the film size is insofar as primary radiation is concerned; there will be "X" number of photons over a four-square centimeter area, or over a forty-square centimeter area. Distribution of primary photons is equal. Distribution of secondary-scatter-photons, however, is unequal. As kVp rises and thickness of irradiated tissue increases, there is an increase in scatter contribution. Increased scatter adversely affects contrast, thus explaining why well-collimated films are of greater diagnostic quality.

There is a definite relationship between area and volume as they relate to collimation. The smaller the area of body surface irradiated, the smaller will be the volume of tissue exposed. If a 10cm x 10cm field area is sufficient for the desired clinical requisites, improper collimation encompassing a 15cm x 15cm field area will yield a volume of irradiated tissue 2.25 times greater than the first example.

Surely this one bit of information should be enough to keep collimator shutters narrowed to the closest possible approximation consistent with imaging objectives.

It is an erroneous belief that tight collimation during an imaging examination will decrease the exposure factors necessary to produce the optimal radiographic result. Not only is this incorrect, the opposite is true. As irradiated areas decrease, exposure values must increase. Scatter radiation contributes substantially to the blackening which occurs on an exposed film. Significant reduction of scatter materially reduces film blackening, necessitating augmented exposure factors to bring density back to normal.

Filtration

Filtration is a very important tool for the x-ray user who wishes to improve diagnostic quality and to lower radiation dosages issued to patients. Filtration affecting the final film result falls into three categories:

(1) Inherent filtration
(2) Added filtration
(3) Tissue of the patient-part undergoing examination.

In this chapter we will be dealing mainly with the first two categories, i.e., filtration sustained by the beam before it reaches the patient. Our primary concern lies with added filtration, particularly that variety accurately described and labelled *Density Equalizing Filtration* (DEF). The purpose of DEF is to homogenize various film densities, rendering the final film result more diagnostic at the same time as lessened radiation dosages are effected. Let us first consider conventional filtration before moving on to the principles and use of DEF.

Filtration: Inherent & Added

Inherent Filtration is that portion comprising the tube and its housing. As discussed in Chapter III, the emergent x-ray beam passes through — in succession — the vacuum within the tube, the glass wall of the tube, insulating oil and the external window known as the tube port.

X-ray physics refers to the amount of reduction in radiation issued as a measurement of *aluminum equivalents*. This is the amount of filtration in aluminum which equals the attenuation produced by the substance(s) concerned. In this instance the inherent filtration between the anode and the tube port generally varies from 0.5mm to 0.9mm aluminum.

Added filtration incorporates those materials interposed between the tube and the film which act as attenuators of the x-ray beam. Manufacturers introduce added filtration to the tube port, commonly 2mm aluminum equivalent. In representative figures the collimator attenuates the beam to an equivalent of 0.75mm aluminum. Adding this figure to the inherent filtration, there is now approximately 3.5mm aluminum equivalent filtration in place between the anode and the patient. Thirty (30) kVp and less wavelength rays are thus effectively removed from the x-ray beam, resulting in a more homogenous beam and lowered radiation to the patient.

The beam is more homogenous because low energy photons have been absorbed by the filtration. The patient receives less radiation because low energy photons, which normally would be absorbed when they encountered the skin and proximal depths of tissue, have been eliminated through the attenuation effect of the filtration. Remember that low energy photons are worthless; they do not reach the film and consequently do not participate in the imaging process. Instead, low energy photons are absorbed by the patient who receives a commensurately increased quota of radiation.

As an x-ray beam undergoes filtration its composition modifies from the original heterogeneous state. The "new" beam contains photons which have comparatively shorter wavelengths, higher kilovoltage and greater penetration than the original beam. This does not mean

USEFUL RANGE OF kVp

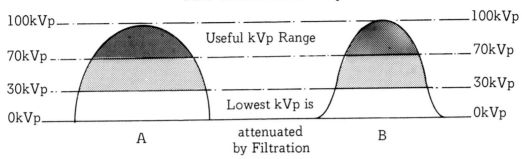

Fig. 7-2 — Schematic illustration of voltage wave forms in relation to kVp. The "peaky" wave form in B is less efficient, yielding fewer high-energy photons. Filtration removes photons from the lower energy range, allowing harder rays to reach the film.

that higher kilovoltage is produced by filtration but it does mean that the selective absorption of lower kilovoltage photons results in a beam containing an increased percentage of the original high kVp photons. This "hardening" of the photon stream causes it to become more difficult to filter, rendering an identical filter relatively less effective. This explains why successive half-value layers become extended as the penetration of a subject proceeds. It also adds further explanation to the fact that the first few centimeters of patient thickness receive more radiation (as well as more backscatter) than deeper structures. The hard rays of higher kilovoltage traverse the patient while the soft rays of lower kilovoltage become absorbed.

The addition of overall filtration necessitates yet another compromise situation in diagnostic radiology. To maintain the same density on the film as occurred without filtration an increase in mAs is necessary. An increase in mAs causes an increased load to be applied to the tube and, of course, places limits upon the use of filters. Whereas an overall filtration of 5mm of aluminum may be eminently practical, 10mm of aluminum could quite easily result in damage to the tube within a brief period. A state of equilibrium must be attained to protect the life of the tube and to protect the life

of the patient.

An increased tube loading via elevated mAs actually decreases the patient "loading." Even though overall filtration brings about an increase in mAs requirements, a corresponding reduction in entrance exposure occurs in this instance due to the consequent attenuation of radiation.

Filtration & Kilovoltage

Kilovoltage is a variable factor in the filtration equation. Lower kilovoltage levels require proportionately greater increases in exposure time to compensate for the attenuation of filtration than do higher kilovoltage levels. (The corollary to this fact is that the use of a high-optimal kVp technique reduces the need for markedly elevated mAs factors.) To obtain the same density reduction at 100 kVp as is obtained at 80 kVp, 40 percent more filtration is required; at 120-125 kVp the amount of filtration necessary is 33 percent more than at 100 kVp.

Step-wedge tests conducted by F. G. Bauer whereby film density was halved through the use of aluminum filtration revealed major discrepancies among nine x-ray installations examined. All units were single-phase fully-rectified with 240 or 415 volts line supply, varying from 15 to 75 amperes. The most inefficient unit required 4.75mm aluminum to halve density while the most efficient unit required

9.25mm aluminum to accomplish the same task. In general the better the intake supply, the better the machine performance at the same kVp setting, therefore the more filtration necessary to obtain a desired result. It is imperative that a good line supply be present if the x-ray user is to gain optimum performance from the generating apparatus.

Resolution is relatively unaffected by filtration. However, contrast does alter noticeably with overall filtration. Because there is more even penetration of an object the contrast level decreases.

To return to the filtration effect upon density and radiation issued, the following figures are pertinent:

At 100 kVp 9.25mm aluminum reduces density by 50 percent;
At 100 kVp 3.17mm aluminum reduces radiation by 50 percent.

It can readily be seen that overall filtration is highly beneficial to the patient at the 100 kVp level, the optimum kVp for spinographic studies with today's imaging equipment. Lower kVp levels require less filtration for a 50 percent reduction in density. For example, at 80 kVp, 6.35mm aluminum reduces density by 50 percent. Techniques utilizing less than 80 kVp have no place in conventional biomechanical imaging examinations of the spine and pelvis.

Fig. 7-2 depicts voltage wave forms of two single-phase x-ray generators and the effect of overall filtration on each one.

The effect of filtration is illustrated in the cross-hatched area between zero kVp and 30 kVp in both diagrams. Radiation from this portion of the cycle is attenuated before it reaches the patient. Fig. 7-2 also illustrates the effects of two different wave-forms. The cycle in Diagram A exhibits a good wave-form while the cycle in B has a "peaky" wave-form. In A there is a greater portion of the cycle above 70 kVp than there is in B. While both machines will produce 100 kVp as read on the kV meter, the machine pro-

ducing the cycle in A will provide a much better output due to its favorable wave-form. In fact, some wave-form patterns are so "peaky" in nature that they resemble a silhouette of the Matterhorn. The x-ray apparatus producing wave-form A similarly will require greater filtration than the machine producing wave-form B because the output is correspondingly greater in the former.

Graded Screens

Graded screens have received considerable attention over many years and they do have their uses. Nevertheless, they are not capable of attenuating radiation or of equalizing the great disparities that may occur in skeletal radiography. Graded screens usually can cope with no greater exposure factors than a 3:1 density differential. This is quite insufficient when, for example, an extremely "wasp-waisted" individual is the subject of a lateral lumbar examination. It is eminently feasible to obtain a single diagnostic quality film extending upwards from the tip of the coccyx as far as — and including — T9 and/or T10. However, specific filtration is necessary to accomplish this task because the great variation in tissue thickness and density occuring in the lateral lumbar examination of a "wasp-waisted" individual necessitates an exposure differential of 17:1 in some instances. This fact alone is reason enough for a discussion of Density Equalizing Filtration (DEF).

Density Equalizing Filtration

Employment of compensating filters was first suggested in 1906 and interest in their use has waxed and waned since that time. Today, application of DEF in conventional radiography is highly recommended; nevertheless, an indifference to its effectiveness is noted repeatedly.

The purpose of DEF is to homogenize various film densities of bodily regions possessing different masses and thicknesses, while lessening radiation exposure to these areas. DEF is additional

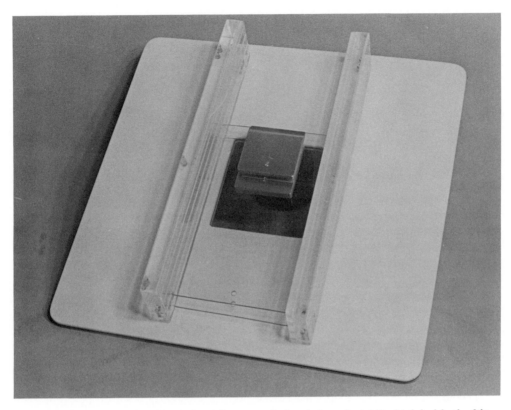

Fig. 7-3 — The laminated plastic-lead-laminated plastic "sandwich" which holds the filters is affixed to the collimator.

filtration which does not require an increase in exposure factors in its use. It filters unnecessary photons from that portion of the beam directed to less dense parts of the patient in a particular exposure. How is this accomplished? It is simply by the introduction of aluminum and/or copper-plus-aluminum filters between the collimator and the film, most often before the beam reaches the patient.

The prominence given to the practical application of DEF in the following pages is done for two reasons:

1. To show what work has been accomplished in this area of diagnostic spinology, and
2. To induce the x-ray user to investigate the possible use of these or similar measures in his/her own spinal imaging procedures.

We believe that several aspects of x-ray usage are the result of custom or tradition; methods have been followed for so long that change is neglected or overlooked. Such is the case with the "spot" view of L5 in the lateral lumbar position. This view is rendered obsolete by the use of DEF, which yields a film of even density throughout the lumbar spine. Considering the proximity of the gonads it is eminently logical to lessen radiation in this area whenever possible. Utilization of filters to bring about this end can make a significant contribution to decremental irradiation of the public.

Composition of DEF

The following filter system has been developed by F. G. Bauer with refinements in design and use evolving over the past fifteen years. There are a total of eight density equalizing filters; five are placed immediately in front of the collimator and three are affixed to the surface of the

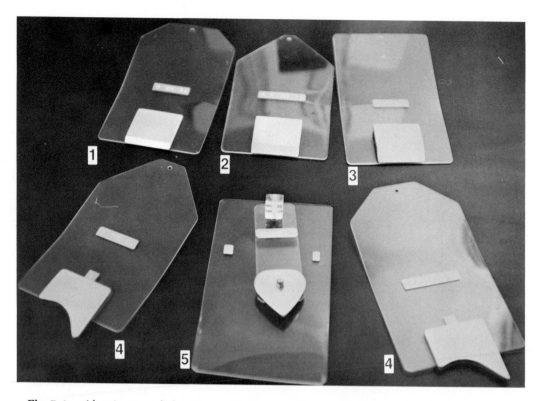

Fig. 7-4 — Aluminum and aluminum-plus-copper filters which are used radiographically to equalize bodily thickness and density differentials.

bucky adjacent to the posterior aspect of the patient's lower cervical spine.

The framework which supports the first five filters is made in the form of a "lead sandwich," 1mm of lead acting as the filling between two pieces of laminated plastic "bread," as seen in Fig. 7-3. Parallel runners termed "filter guides" have four tracks which allow for the insertion and placement of the filters. The window in the support plate is proportioned so that it is just large enough for the x-ray beam to cover the area of the largest cassette used. This assists in reducing the effects of any minor tube leak. The framework is mounted to the front of the collimator in one of two ways. For permanent installation it is simply attached by screws. For convertible use runners can be attached to the lead sandwich and a reciprocal track mounted on the collimator.

The filters (Fig. 7-4) are mounted onto an unbreakable, flexible clear acrylic sheet (commercially known as "Lexan") which has been given a "set." The slight deflection in the acrylic exerts enough force to enable any of the filters to be retained at any point along the tracks without the installation of a specific restraining mechanism.

Filters 1, 2 and 3 are of aluminum construction, their respective thicknesses being 3mm, 4mm and 6mm aluminum. All filters exhibit a high degree of workmanship to ensure consistency of radiographic results. The inferior ends of these three filters are brought to a fine wedge taper which prevents the film viewer from perceiving the presence of filtration in any normal circumstance. These filters are used in A-P Cervicothoracic and Lateral Lumbar examinations, details of their implementation to follow shortly.

Filter 4 is a lung filter, used to lessen part of the great exposure differential existing between L5 and T11 or T12. The curved shape follows the path of the diaphragm across the lateral lumbar film. The filter is composed of 1.5mm aluminum on each side of an 0.5mm copper core. Aluminum absorbs characteristic radiation which is produced by copper and so the aluminum is placed on the patient side of the filter in normal circumstances. Because this filter is reversible, aluminum is on the patient side of the copper whether the patient's left or right side is directed towards the bucky.

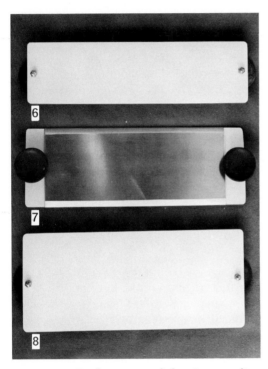

Fig. 7-5 — Bucky-mounted density equalizing filters for the mid-to-lower cervical spine.

Filter 5 is of the same material as filter 4, heart-shaped and called a back-scatter filter. Its heart shape and swing arm mounting allow it to be positioned over the posterior portion of the spinous processes in the cervical and lumbar spines irrespective of the shape of the patient's curve. If desired, it also can be employed as a thyroid filter in the lateral cervical view.

Filters 6, 7 and 8 (Fig. 7-5) are density equalizing filters for the mid-to-lower cervical spine. These filters are placed behind the patient to attain the greatest diagnostic improvement possible, part of which results from the lessened contribution of scatter radiation. There is no reduction of patient dosage with the use of these filters. However, the adoption of an optimal kVp technique, long FFD, and the use of other filtration ensures that the cervicothoracic area receives a minimal exposure dose.

Each filter is 20cm across, from lateral margin to lateral margin, the height and thickness of aluminum varying per filter. Filter 6 is 7cm in height, the aluminum being 3mm in thickness. Filter 7 is 9cm in height and 4mm aluminum in thickness. The thickness of filter 8 is the same as the preceding one while the height is increased to 11cm. The last filter is used to aid in visualization of an individual with a particularly long and slender neck, or in conjunction with the moving-jaw technique. Aluminum is bonded to laminated plastic in each of these three filters, the superior and inferior portions of the aluminum tapered evenly to guarantee invisibility upon the final film result. Small rubber suction cups allow the filters to be positioned easily or realigned as required.

A-P Cervicothoracic Spine

An elongated cervical film, extending from base of occiput to the approximate level of the tenth Thoracic vertebrae possesses additional information that is most helpful in biomechanical evaluation of the patient. The radiation-laden and archaic 14" x 36" (35cm x 91cm) "full-spine" film suffers from excessive magnification, distortion and exposure dose; the 8" x 10" (20cm x 25cm) film has none of these disadvantages but it often is inadequate in extent. To obviate the necessity for an A-P Thoracic view the cervical and thoracic regions can be investigated — in the antero-posterior direction — by one 7" x 17" (18cm x 43cm) exposure.

The radiographs in Fig. 7-6 offer a comparison between filtration and non-filtration. The same patient is shown in each radiograph, A being correctly filtered while B is unfiltered.

The exposure should be calculated to produce the correct density from T4 or T5 to T10. Superior to T4/5 filtration is necessary to homogenize the great density disparities which normally would occur in a film of this region. Filters 1, 2 and 3 are used, either singly or in combination. With the 100 kVp technique the superior portion of the film requires 10mm to 12mm of filtration, depending of course on patient thickness. Filtration is positioned so that its full breadth is present at the approximate level of T2 while the inferior bevelled edge(s) extend to T4/5.

Now either filter 6, 7 or 8 is placed behind the upright patient, being affixed to the bucky front. Without this filter C5-T2 would remain overexposed. Eighty (80) percent of radiation already has been eliminated by other filtration so installing this filter between the patient and the film is quite reasonable.

The moving-jaw technique requires a filter of greater height than the stationary open-mouth technique. This is because the superior border of the filter is level with the inferior portion of the closed jaw in the moving-jaw procedure. The jaw is open in the latter procedure, requiring less compensating filtration for the area covered by the inferior mandibular mass.

A-P Thoracic Spine

Taking a 43cm (17″) exposure of the thoracic spine generally necessitates DEF over the superior portion of the film. Approximately 6mm aluminum extending inferiorly to T4/5 is sufficient in the unattainable yet ubiquitous "average" man. In regard to aged patients, DEF should not extend beneath the T3/4 level. The objective is to avoid filtering the aortic arch, a structure which may become sclerotic in advancing years.

A-P Lumbosacral Spine

Filtration generally is unnecessary unless a very thin patient is being examined, in which case the number 1 filter containing 3mm of A1. is used. The filter is inserted in the filter guides so that it extends coverage from the cephalic aspect of the pelvis upwards to the superior film border.

Lateral Cervical Spine

Biomechanical considerations obligate mention of general positioning technique for lateral views of any spinal area. If a lateral cervical film is taken in the sitting position there is an exaggeration of the normal cervical lordosis as compared to the result obtained in a standing film. If the lateral lumbar examination is conducted in the recumbent position the usual lumbar lordosis is reduced, particularly if the hips and knees are flexed. There often will be an alteration in spinal configuration between recumbent, sitting and standing lateral spinal films. The apex of a scoliotic curvature should be placed towards the film to permit viewing into the convexity of the curve. Herein, all reference to positioning denotes the standing position.

No wedge filters are necessary in the lateral cervical spine examination. The heart-shaped number 5 filter is positioned so that it is superimposed over the posterior neck surface to a depth of approximately 12mm (1/2″). This improves diagnostic value and reduces scatter radiation derived from posterior cervical musculature.

Another use for this filter is to shield the thyroid gland. This may be the preferred method of utilization if the patient being examined has undergone previous extensive imaging examinations or if the patient is a youth.

Lateral Thoracic Spine

The upper thoracic region often is obscured by both shoulders, requiring a "swimmer's" view to discern this area.

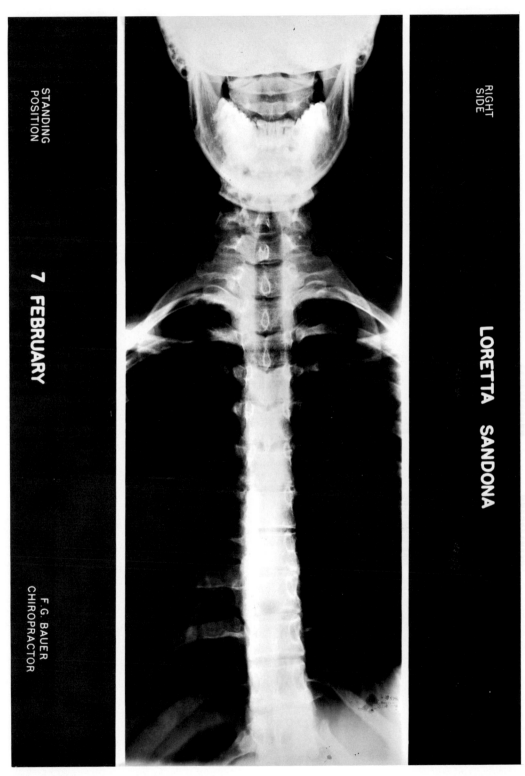

STANDING POSITION

7 FEBRUARY

F. G. BAUER
CHIROPRACTOR

RIGHT SIDE

LORETTA SANDONA

Fig. 7-6-A

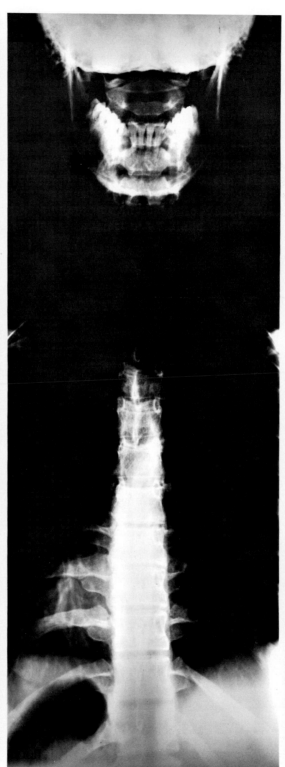
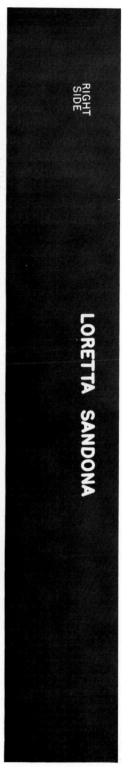

STANDING POSITION

7 FEBRUARY

F. G. BAUER
CHIROPRACTOR

RIGHT SIDE

LORETTA SANDONA

Fig. 7-6-B

The usual lateral thoracic view simply omits the upper thoracic vertebrae. An improved radiographic result can be obtained with the aid of DEF. Insert one of filters 1 through 3 from the inferior end of the filter guides, sliding upwards as far as T4 or T5. The thickness of aluminum varies from 3mm to 6mm depending on the thoracic physique of a given individual. A reliable rule of thumb for DEF directs that more filtration is needed with solidly built, well muscled individuals because exposure factors are higher for this group. Remember that exposure factors are to be calculated from the most dense area to be projected onto the film; density in more radiolucent areas needs to be reduced with DEF. Computation is based upon 9.5mm Al. reducing the density of the film by 50 percent at 100 kVp.

Lateral Lumbar Spine, Including Sacrum and Coccyx

A visual representation of filtration benefits in the lateral lumbar view is included in the "Practical Perspective" accompanying this chapter.

Lateral lumbar views were frequently taken on 8" x 10" films. These views are merely large spot films, falling far short of the information potential available from this area. The ideal film size in such situations is the 7" x 17" (18cm x 43cm) film and the lateral view may even be collimated to a useful width of 6" (15cm) in 99 percent of examination. Strict collimation is recommended particularly to reduce unnecessary radiation to the patient and to minimize scatter radiation which, in this area, contributes amply to the formation of fog. The 7" x 17" film size accommodates two or three of the lowest thoracic vertebrae, all lumbar vertebrae and the entire sacrum and coccyx, furnishing a great deal of information upon a relatively small area of film. We disagree with the long standing radiologic practice of taking several views in a standard lumbar imaging examination. This pro-

cedure often includes an A-P lumbar spine, lateral lumbar spine, lateral lumbar spot view, and bilateral oblique lumbar spines. Sometimes an A-P or P-A sacral film also is incorporated into the examination. Such procedures certainly invest the patient with a powerful exposure dose, quite often needlessly. The basic examination we recommend for the lumbar area is A-P and lateral lumbar spine films, especially for children and adult males and females of reproductive potential, followed by additional views if initial findings indicate they are necessary.

Professor K. Morgan is an eminent authority on radiation and its effects. As long ago as 1971 Dr. Morgan declared that diagnostic x-ray exposure in America could be reduced to one-tenth of its present amount without any loss of benefits. One of the ways to reduce this radiation exposure is by eliminating an exhaustive examination procedure when a simpler one will suffice.

Begin applying DEF in the lateral lumbar examination by inserting the diaphragmatic filter number 4 so that it approximates the level of the diaphragm. This is found most usually to be aligned at the superior plate of the first lumbar vertebral body or partially upwards upon T12. This region may appear completely black in radiographic films due to total penetration of the subject. To obtain an even film density the lung field area seen above the diaphragm requires less than six percent of the radiation necessary for proper exposure at the level of the L5 disc. Install filter 5, the heart-shaped model, so that it overlies the posterior half of the lumbar spinous processes. This measurably reduces the over-penetration which characteristically occurs in the spinouses, and lessens backscatter originating from the heavy, posterior spinal musculature. The shape and maneuverability of the filter accommodates hyperlordotic or hypolordotic lumbar spines; the point of the "heart" faces upwards as the filter turns upon its axis. The spinous processes are involved in the positioning procedure for a lateral lumbar examination — the patient is placed so that the tip of L4 spinous process is approximately 2.5cm (1") anterior to the collimated rear margin of the film. Almost all patients fit this positioning procedure; however, the size of a patient and his/her lumbar lordotic configuration are variable factors. The third filter to be positioned is one of the wedge filters, being 3mm, 4mm or 6mm Al. in thickness. This filtration is superimposed over the entire upper portion of the film, extending inferiorly so that the bevelled end reaches the upper aspect of the iliac crests. The amount of filtration required to equalize density above L5 depends upon the individual being examined. A parallel-waisted person would need no more than 3mm DEF; a moderate figure would require 4mm DEF; and a full-hipped, wasp-waisted woman may require 6mm filtration. The use of the three filters described in the preceding paragraphs will reduce the overall radiation exposure of the entire field by no less than 50 percent and, as stated previously, render the L5 "spot" film altogether superfluous. Concurrently the diagnostic quality of the film will improve markedly. DEF makes a most significant contribution to decreased radiation exposure levels in lateral lumbar imaging procedures. At best, omission of filtration is thoughtless; at worst, it borders on negligence.

To summarize, with particular reference to the lateral lumbar view, DEF balances film densities. The exposure is set for the area of most difficult penetration while lesser areas are selectively filtered. No increase in exposure factors is required. There definitely is an increase in film area transformed into real diagnostic worth.

Considerations in Lumbar Spinology

An important factor in preparing for a lateral lumbar exposure is to determine which side of the standing patient should be placed against the bucky front. Should any degree of scoliotic curvature be present there is only one side that can be positioned against the bucky for optimal viewing, and that is the side of convexity. Ideally, in order to obtain the most favorable and precise alignment of superior and inferior vertebral body plates, and consequent perception of intervertebral disc spacing, the vertebral bodies would need to be aligned in an arc conforming with the periphery of an imaginary wheel. The center — or hub — of this wheel is the focal spot and the rim is the vertebral column of the individual being examined. While it is not always possible to attain this perfection it is at least possible to position a patient according to the ideal-arc precept. That is the concept which dictates the placement of the side of convexity towards the film.

How does one determine the scoliotic disposition of a patient? The most accurate method is to execute the A-P lumbar spinographic examination, develop the film and review it briefly prior to undertaking the lateral examination. This time-conscious individual will note that this method involves an additional development process, consuming valuable time. It is true that one extra film processing cycle is necessary for manual, deep-tank installations. (The time differential is minimal for installations utilizing automatic processing.) There is only one additional processing cycle for manual facilities because the lateral lumbar spine film, once exposed, can be retained and developed with the films of the next patient. For example, let us suppose six patients are to receive radiological examinations during morning office hours, all involving a lumbar spine examination. The first patient has an anteriorposterior lumbar spine exposure and the x-ray user processes this film prior to taking the lateral lumbar spine exposure. The lateral film is retained, to be developed with the next set of films requiring processing. Thus, seven processing procedures are necessary for six examinations. A few moments have been consumed while achieving enhanced film results. A further advantage to developing the anteriorposterior lumbar spine film first concerns the positioning of the diaphragmatic filter number 4. The position of the typical diaphragm does not alter significantly. Nevertheless, minor vari-

ations do occur in the level at which the diaphragm partitions the torso. To determine the exact height of the diaphragm, consult the processed anteriorposterior film for guidance. The initial review of this film provides direction for placing number 4 filter, plus communicating which side of the patient will rest against the bucky. The configuration of filter number 4 renders it readily reversible, convenient to use with either left side or right side application.

Practical Perspective

BEAM REDUCTION WITH ADDITIONAL AL FILTRATION AT 100 kVp

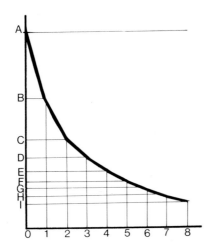

A 100% Normal operating condition
   (Inherent filtration, 2mm added
   AL in Port & Collimator)
B 66.6% 2mm AL in front of Collimator
C 44.4% 4mm " " " "
D 36.1% 6mm " " " "
E 27.8% 8mm " " " "
F 23.2% 10mm " " " "
G 18.7% 12mm " " " "
H 15.2% 14mm " " " "
I 12.2% 16mm " " " "
   Half value thickness at 100 kVp = 3.3mm added AL
   Half value thickness at 80 kVp = 2.5mm added AL

The graph plots the reduction of radiation which occurs as a result of attenuating the x-ray beam with collimator-mounted aluminum filtration. Tests conducted by the radiation branch of the Health Commission of New South Wales found that the HVL of the subject x-ray machine was 3.3mm added AL at 100 kVp and 2.5mm added AL at 80 kVp. This information provided the basis for the preparation of the chart. The amount of radiation at point A is the total quantity of radiation present under normal operating conditions. The addition of 2mm of AL reduces the radiation exposure to two-thirds of its former intensity. Similarly, 6mm of AL reduces the radiation exposure to nearly one-third of its original value.

Note that as the beam "hardens" each 2mm increment of added AL has less effect than the previous addition. Soft rays are easily attenuated, rendering the first layers of AL more effective than succeeding thicknesses.

Comparing the percentages of radiation reduction at points A throught I to the millimetric thicknesses of AL utilized, illustrates why density equalizing filtration is so successful in reducing the radiation exposures given to patients in everyday clinical situations.

Practical Perspective

COLLIMATOR ALIGNMENT

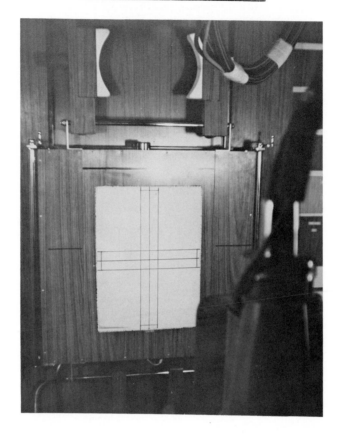

The step-by-step procedures for aligning a collimator are included in the text in "Collimator Alignment." The purpose here is to give a brief review of this topic. The photograph is taken from a position adjacent to the x-ray tube, showing a high speed intensifying screen affixed to a wall bucky. Heavy lines are marked on the screen to assist alignment procedures conducted in semi-darkness.

The central ray of the x-ray tube must be at right angles to the bucky face. It is easy to surmise that service personnel have done their job perfectly but this is not always the case. The x-ray user can readily check tube-bucky alignment to satisfy himself as to its correctness.

Whether the x-ray machine tracks are situated on the ceiling or on the floor, remember that they must remain perpendicular to the bucky. The ideal installation is one which allows for the tracks to be shifted medially or laterally throughout their length.

To check the alignment of the x-ray tube and its stand, position the tube as far away from the bucky as possible on the tracks. Allow the light beam to be opened slightly in the vertical direction, the upright shutters creating a slit of light directed to the center of the bucky face. As the tube is moved forward this band of light will become smaller but it should remain centered in the middle of the focused area during its entire traveling distance.

Chapter **8**

Patient Stabilization & Gonadal Protection

Always position the patient accurately. Immobilizing devices should be used when necessary and practicable. If the exposure has to be repeated, the radiation to the patient is doubled.

K.C. Clark, *Positioning in Radiography*, p. 778, Ninth Edition, Volume 2, Published for Ilford by Wm. Heinman, 1973.

In 1975 a United States government publication (GONAD SHIELDING IN DIAGNOSTIC RADIOLOGY, DHEW PUBLICATION (FDA) 75-8024) stoutly advocated utilization of gonadal shielding:

"On a national scale, the conscientious use of gonad shields in appropriate diagnostic examinations will produce a significant reduction in the number of potentially deleterious mutations which would otherwise be expressed in future generations. It is the cumulative nature of these genetic changes distributed over succeeding generations that makes the use of gonad shielding a public health concern."

This same manifesto declared that testicular shielding techniques were "better established" than protective measures for ovarian shielding. The authors declare:

"It may be possible for examining physicians to use ovarian shielding during selected views in some examinations, but these techniques have not as yet been well established."

Practical techniques for the deployment of testicular and ovarian shielding had indeed been well established by concerned Australian practitioners, following developments in this field by F. G. Bauer during the late 1960's and early 1970's. This chapter deals with these developments, practical measures to ensure gonadal protection, in conjunction with methods to obtain patient immobilization.

Steadying Devices

The term *unsharpness* has a ring of persecuted grammar to it; however, it is a familiar and aptly applied descriptive label, one which defines the status of a radiograph in a single word. Several kinds of unsharpness exist including geometric, screen, absorption, motion and parallax unsharpness. Motion unsharpness is our present concern.

During an imaging exposure no disruptive movement should occur to the patient or to the radiographic equipment. Situations where movement does occur result in unsharpness or, simply, blurring of the film. Diagnostic radiology is no different than general photography in this aspect: movement results in the formation of a blurred picture.

Kinetic factors contributing to blurring include:

(1) film movement, and
(2) anode movement.

Film movement refers to bucky shudder, vibration or any of the innumerable varieties of positional shifts which may occur within the bucky and its supportive framework. Because the film — in the cassette — becomes an integral part of the bucky structure during the time of the exposure, the film will deviate from its normal position to the same degree as the bucky arrangement deviates from its normal position. This problem is entirely mechanical in nature and a complete review of the subject is found in Chapter IV.

Anode movement is any motion which occurs beyond the expected rotation of the anode around its own stem. It is of lesser magnitude than film movement but it does contribute to unsharpness. The two principal causes of anode movement are:

(a) earth tremors, and
(b) faulty floor support.

Nature's earth tremors do not bear upon the results obtained in the usual radiographic installation. On the other hand, man-made earth tremors must be considered in any discussion of anode movement. Passing trains and heavy vehicular traffic in urban or other settled areas can, at times, shake the foundation of a building. Because the x-ray tube generally is attached to the unit by way of an extended column, the effects of a tremorous building may be magnified.

It is clear that floor support must be sufficient to maintain the entire x-ray apparatus in an immobile state. This is more easily accomplished in a concrete floor structure than in a wooden building. Because a wooden beamed floor is more liable to vibrate than a concrete platform, it should be checked for movement. This can be done with the aid of a wide-mouthed glass or a saucer of water, as described at length in Practical Perspective, for establishing bucky and tube stability.

Place a shallow dish of water on top of the x-ray tube and have someone walk around the room; it is even beneficial to have someone walk around in adjacent rooms. If any ripples form on the liquid in the saucer there is tube movement and consequently, anode movement. This same test also is recommended when checking for man-made earth tremors.

The installation of additional posts or other supportive foundation buttressing must be carried out where required if the x-ray user hopes to achieve optimal results.

Patient movement is much more common than is generally realized, especially accompanying the upright position, where the clinician seeks information of a biomechanical nature in an imaging examination. Since it is virtually impossible for an individual to stand absolutely still, it is necessary to enlist the aid of stabilizing accessories, particularly in the area of interest.

Patient movement can be placed in one of two categories:

(a) involuntary movement involving voluntary muscles, and
(b) involuntary movement involving involuntary muscles.

It is fortunate that involuntary movement of involuntary muscles does not noticeably hinder the spinographic study for it cannot be eliminated in any event. Occasionally patients are anxious and somewhat unsettled during an examination. A calm, professional approach to duties effects the most satisfactory response from the patient. If the x-ray user is dashing and darting about breathlessly, or displaying a brusque manner, or conveying an overly familiar and causal air, the patient is unlikely to be serene and relaxed. The x-ray user must remember that the patient is not usually familiar with procedures that are encountered every day in a radiographic department, and that lessened patient movement will ensue if imaging activities are directed at the patient's welfare instead of the operator's gratification.

The Bilateral Compression Band (BCB)

Involuntary movement involving voluntary muscles can be mitigated by employing *patient steadying devices*. A most useful patient steadying device is the *bilateral compression band* (BCB) designed by F. G. Bauer as an adjunct in the upright lumbar and pelvic imaging examination. Unilateral compression devices have been used for many years, for recumbent and erect views. Their weakness is that radiographic distortion of relevant trunk structures may occur due to the unequal application of compression.

The bucky-mounted BCB essentially comprises two metal shafts and a broad band, 14″ (35cm) in height. (Refer to Fig. 8-5 through 8-8 for illustrations of the bilateral compression band, used in conjunction with the gonadal shielding.) The metal shafts are aligned vertically, affixed at the lateral margins of the bucky and equipped with spring-locked winders which allow the band to be tensioned against the area of interest. The band is made of a sturdy fabric or vinyl material with minimal stretch deformity characteristics. If, for example, an A-P Lumbar visualization is to be done, the patient stands back-to-bucky in the usual manner. The x-ray user inserts the band borders into the metal shafts and both sides are tightened simultaneously. This method of compression does not apply any torsion to the body and so no rotational deviation occurs.

Studies done with-and-without the BCB reveal that no distortion is introduced to the patient through its use. Leg deficiencies, postural deviations and biomechanical disrelationships are revealed in a patient constrained by the BCB with the same clarity as they are revealed in a free-standing individual. In fact, often the "compressed" patient yields a more diagnostically acceptable result. The two radiographs shown in Fig. 8-1 present an example confirming this statement. Both films are of the same individual. The patient is free-standing in 8-1 A while in 8-1 B he is restrained within the BCB. No change in the scoliotic pattern is evident in B and the diagnostic quality of the film is improved.

There are several reasons for the improved final film result with compression. Firstly, the individual is immobile. Secondly, the patient thickness is reduced due to the compression effect; this in itself tends to improve the diagnostic quality. Thirdly, the decreased thickness lessens scatter radiation. In summation, everyone benefits from improved diagnostic quality while the patient receives a further ancillary advantage: lessened radiation. Decreased patient thickness means that less mAs has to be used, other factors remaining equal, thereby reducing the dose received.

With obese patients the BCB considerably reduces the entrance dose of radiation by reducing the object thickness. There have been instances with extremely obese patients where radiation reduction has approached 50 percent. The aim in examining the obese patient is not only to obtain stabilization but to obtain compression as well. The BCB tension will be in excess of the normal requirements for steadying only.

It must be remembered that there is a limit to the amount of compression which can be exerted against any patient, and this fact becomes more consequential in dealing with the obese. An intemperate

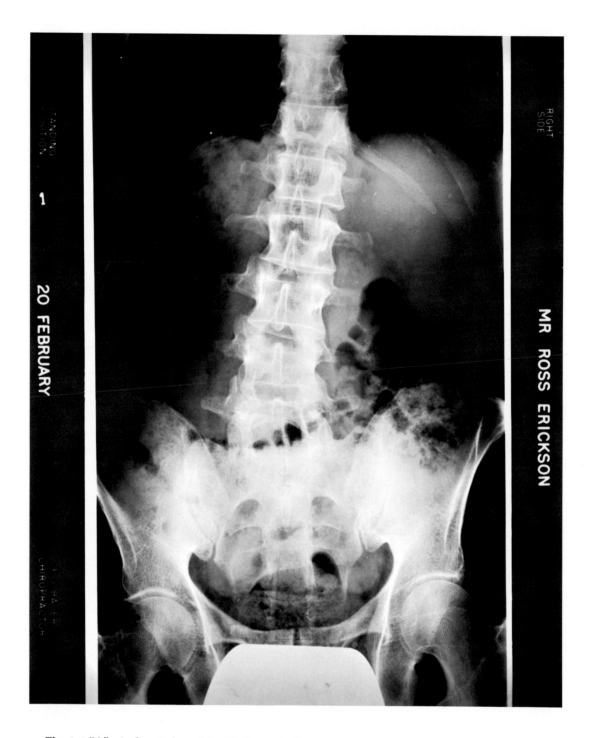

Fig. 8-1 "A" - In fig. A the subject is free standing.

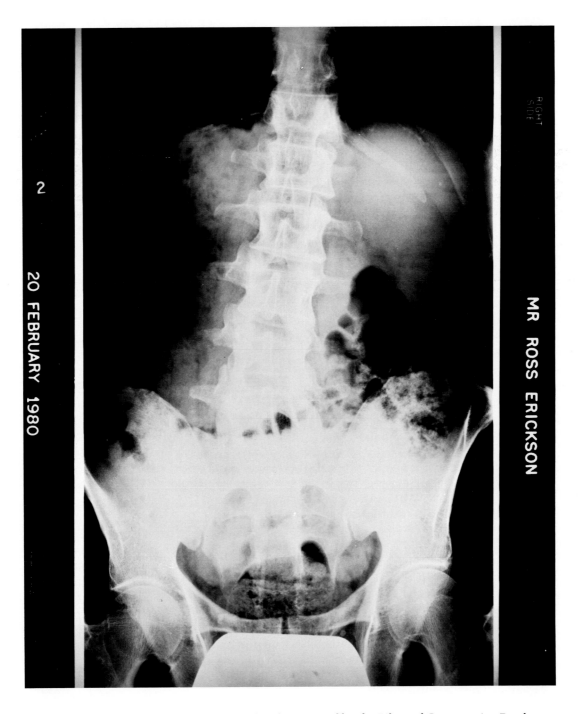

Fig. 8-1 "B" - In B the subject is supported and restrained by the Bilateral Compression Band. No change in the Scoliotic Pattern occurs through the use of the· BCB.

endeavor to compress the patient will cause increasing pressure against the bucky front. This pressure can cause the bucky front to yield inwardly, interfering with the travel of the grid and resulting in a slowing down or even a complete halt in grid movement.

The material used in fronting the bucky is important to the final radiographic result. The structure must be strong enough to allow unimpeded grid travel while at the same time being light enough to attenuate minimal amounts of radiation. Reinforcing the lateral portions of the bucky front adds stability to the overall structure and does not interfere with the imaging area.

The bucky front commonly is faced with a synthetic resin or plastic material; "Bakelite" is one such commercial product. Laminated plastic also is used, as is a comparatively recent market arrival containing graphite. Irrespective of material chosen, perform several "test runs" with the grid travelling across the bucky while a co-worker is subjected to various tensions from the BCB. Observation will determine whether grid travel is proceeding normally.

The broad band is well suited for A-P Thoracic views due to the lengthy section of torso visualized. Application of the BCB in this instance is similar to its use in A-P Lumbar-Pelvic imaging examinations. While there is little compressibility in lateral Thoracolumbosacral investigations the BCB is used to great advantage in obtaining immobilization. In those instances where a patient is somewhat unsteady a triangular block fashioned from polystyrene material approximately 2" (5cm) thick can be used in conjunction with the BCB to arrest any remaining movement. This block fits into the triangle created by the patient's relevant posterior surface, the bucky front and the inner surface of the compression band.

Cervical Head-Steadiers

In the cervical region of the spine stabilization is afforded through the use of polystyrene head-steadiers. The blocks employed for support in lateral cervical visualizations (Fig. 8-2) are produced in various depths to fit patients of all sizes and ages. These blocks replace the air space between the bucky front and the lateral aspect of the patient's head. Their purpose is to prevent patient movement while maintaining the head in a neutral position. The series of photographs in Fig. 8-3 show the cervical steadiers in position. First the steadier is employed on its own, then in conjunction with a narrow support band. The patient is next seen with the correct cervical steadier for her conformation, followed by two incorrectly-sized steadiers, one allowing tube-side lateral cervical flexion and the other allowing film-side lateral cervical flexion.

The bucky side of the steadier is flat; it rests evenly against the bucky while the supportive plane maintains a 90° angle to the bucky front. The head side of the steadier is concave, designed to accommodate the patient's head immediately superior to the external ear. The concavity is such that it is somewhat too concave to fit the contour of the head. The result is a 2-point cranial contact, anterior and posterior in location.

These steadiers are most helpful in reducing patient movement among the aged, the infirm and the restless young as well as the seemingly stable patients who make up the majority of a conventional practice. It does not take a great deal of cranial movement to create unsharpness in the cervical area. The steadiers can be used individually or in the preferred manner, i.e., in combination with a compression band. Applied on its own, the patient simply uses slight pressure of his/her head to maintain the steadier in position. The slight increase in muscular hypertonicity aids in arresting tremulous patient movement. Applied in conjunction with a compression band, stabilization is even more

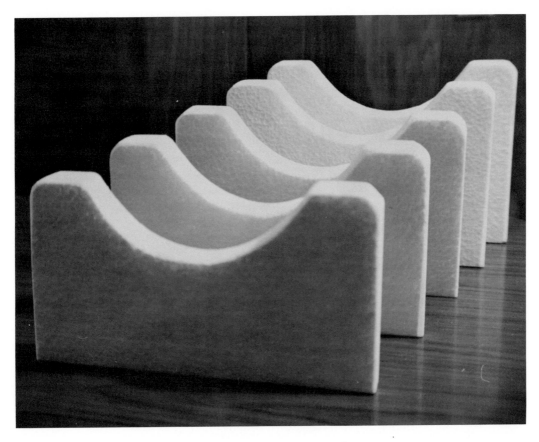

Fig. 8-2 — A set of head-steadiers for use in lateral cervical exposures.

complete. A narrow band of 2″ (5cm) breadth secures the patient's head in position once the correct size steadier has been positioned.

For A-P Cervical visualizations small blocks — made of the same polystyrene material — should be used to fit into the space between the bucky and the patient's head. The narrow compression band is used once again, contacting the patient across the forehead. The blocks will of necessity be of differing sizes since patients' heads are varying distances from the upright bucky.

If the bucky can be inclined, its superior portion tilting forward, the need for blocks is obviated. Head clamps are available commercially and they function well in promoting stability. For all clinicians interested in biomechanical integrity during imaging examinations, an im-

portant factor to keep in mind is that of naturalness. All the preceding restraining measures allow a patient to retain his/her "normal" posture, even if this posture is "abnormal." A steadying device must be applied with prudence and accuracy so that no "correction" of osseous structures ensues.

Supplementary Suggestions

Lateral lumbar exposures conducted in the upright position gain additional stability from the use of a stabilizing staff (SS). The SS is placed in front of the patient, whose hands are placed on top of it. The arms are outstretched and relaxed, resting lightly on the SS. Care must be taken so that no more than half of the arm's weight rests on this support; the lumbar lordosis may be accentuated if excessive weight is applied. The SS does

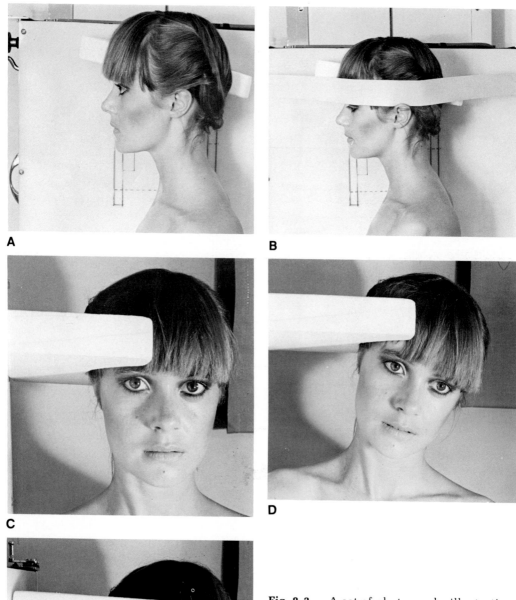

A

B

C

D

E

Fig. 8-3 — A set of photographs illustrating:
— The cervical head-steadier in position (A)
and complemented by a narrow bilateral compression band (B).
The correct steadier is employed (C) in comparison to one allowing tube-side lateral
cervical flexion (D) and one allowing film-side lateral cervical flexion (E).

ensure that the arms do not remain within any portion of the field of view, nor do they receive any unnecessary radiation, always a matter of significance.

Although breathing normally is accomplished subconsciously, respiratory movements can be altered or modified for short periods. Any area of interest removed from the rib cage will gain additional sharpness if breathing is voluntarily arrested; this also applies to the A-P Thoracic spine. Lateral Thoracic visualizations are bettered by allowing quiet, unforced breathing; this tends towards a degree of obliteration of the ribs.

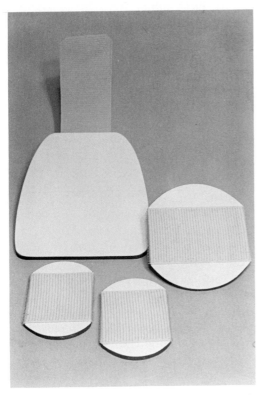

Fig. 8-4 — Set of gonadal shields. Female shields are shown with the patient-side of each shield facing upwards. Velcro material allows shields to be readily attached to the pads of the BCB.

Gonadal Protection

Any person having reproductive potential should be provided with gonadal shielding if the area of the imaging examination includes or is in close proximity to the gonads. The only exception to this dictum occurs when shielding may encroach upon the field of clinical interest; this circumstance prevails much less frequently than is commonly held to be true, especially in conventional osseous imaging of the lumbar spine and pelvis. The four shields used in conjunction with the BCB are pictured in Fig. 8-4. The female shields are turned face-up to show the velcro attachment bands.

Male and female gonads are particularly susceptible to ionizing radiation. Because male gonads reside in such close proximity to the skin surface they enjoy almost none of the protection offered by surrounding tissue. The ovaries are located relatively centrally within the body, generally encircled by approximately 4″ (10cm) of pelvic tissue which provides worthwhile attenuation of radiation. Only a small portion of the total skin dose will ever reach the ovaries, an advantage that does nothing to reduce the imperative for proper shielding.

Science tells us that genetic effects may outweigh the somatic effects of x-ray radiation. Aside from gonadal considerations the in utero embryo would receive the most severe damage. The possible inimical effects of diagnostic level exposures, especially those occurring in the first trimester of pregnancy, are to be avoided at all times.

To assure at least some degree of safety, imaging examinations of a reproductive aged female should be conducted only within the confines of the *Ten-Day Rule*, which states:

> *"Irradiation of the lower abdomen and pelvis of a woman of reproductive age should be confined to the ten days following the first day of the last menstrual period."*

Mechanical and/or chemical contraceptive measures are not foolproof, as any number of disgruntled individuals will attest. The only sure way to avoid the possibility of exposing a pregnant female is to follow the dictates of the Ten-Day Rule. Obviously, if a female has had a hysterectomy, a tubal ligation or is sterile for some other reason the Ten-Day Rule ceases to be of relevance. If a woman is taking an oral contraceptive, most likely it will be safe to conduct a radio-diagnostic examination.

Male Gonadal Protection

When one remembers how many films have been reviewed over a period of several years, recalling how few of these films revealed any gonadal protection, it would be logical to assume that no efforts have been made toward shielding the gonads. This is indeed an understandable though false impression; several varieties of male gonadal safeguards have been developed. A general outline includes the following types:

    I. Contact Shields -
      (A) Flat
      (B) Shaped

    II. Shadow Shields -
      (A) "Free-Standing"
      (B) Machine Mounted

Contact shields are those varieties which rest against the gonads, directly or indirectly. Since many Lumbosacropelvic films are done in the recumbent position (erroneously in our opinion, since bio-mechanical factors often are altered or distorted with a recumbent view) flat contact shields can be rested or taped above the gonads in the A-P view. Shaped contact shields are used on their own or can be installed within briefs which resemble jockey shorts or athletic supporters. These pouch-like protectors provide coverage for additional views but they do require regular care if hygienic standards are to be maintained.

Free-standing shadow shields are mounted on a support stand which is placed on the tabletop in a recumbent examination or on the floor between the x-ray machine and the patient in an upright examination. Machine mounted shadow shields are affixed to the unit, interposed between collimator and patient, allowing the resultant shadow to overlie the gonads.

The gonadal shielding developed by F. G. Bauer fits into the category of "flat, contact shields" (Fig. 8-5). The male shield is 15cm (6″) long, 12cm (4½″) wide at its broadest point and designed so that all corners are well-rounded. The protective lead is 3mm thick, interposed between laminated plastic layers which insure the structural integrity of the shield.

A 5cm (2″) piece of velcro hook extends above the superior end of the shield. This velcro hook adheres to the velcro pad which is situated on the anterior surface of the BCB. This form of gonadal shielding is easily positioned, is economical in cost, is quite comfortable and non-embarrassing for the patient.

The U.S. government publication (DHEW 75-8024) quoted at the beginning of this chapter states that, "the dose reduction may approach 95%" when shields of 0.5mm lead are utilized. Shields of 3mm lead provide protection in the order of 99 percent, the minimal radiation reaching the gonads being mainly scatter.

In the imaging examination of the Lumbo-sacropelvic region — or portion thereof — an A-P erect view entails patient-positioning with stabilization provided by the BCB. Suppose that the collimated lower limit of the film extends 5mm below the inferior aspect of the ischium. The gonadal shield should be positioned so that 1cm of its upper surface is visible on the film. Such positioning proves that shielding was used but it does not inter-fere with any osseous structures in the region of the bony pelvis. For lateral and oblique projections (Fig. 8-6) the gonadal shield is again attached to the velcro insert of the BCB, situated so that it appears on the inferior aspect of the film.

The erect Lumbosacropelvic exami-nation receives advantages in positioning that do not accrue to recumbent tech-niques. Due to the law of gravity and the manner in which the male gonads are suspended, the testicles are generally out of the useful field in most views. To take advantage of this fortunate situation under-pants must not be "hitched-up"; this procedure simply draws the gonads upwards, towards or into the area of interest. The ideal method is to have the patient remove his undershorts prior to the imaging examination, if desired donning a patient gown for modesty's sake. If undershorts are not removed they should be lowered at least enough to allow the gonads to assume the "free-fall" position.

Female Gonadal Protection

Real and imagined "clinical complexities" have prevented widespread adoption of gonadal shielding in the female. Some crude attempts at such shielding have nearly eradicated the sacrum, coccyx and pelvis from the resulting film. With a modicum of care there is no reason why maximum information content cannot be obtained in conjunction with minimal radiation issued to the ovaries.

The gonadal shields for females are quite similar to the male variety — 3mm thickness lead interposed between layers of plastic laminate and backed with velcro for attachment to the BCB. The shields used in A-P visualizations (Fig. 8-7) are 7cm and 5.5 cm wide (approximately 2.7" x 2"), the narrow ends rounded off to lessen unnecessary tissue overlay. Obviously, a pair of shields must be employed so that both ovaries are protected.

Examination of the Lumbosacropelvic region in the lateral position requires a single, larger shield to shade both ovaries (Fig. 8-8). This shield is of the same structure as the others and nearly the same shape as the small A-P female models; however, it is noticeably larger, spanning 9.5cm (3-3/4").

As evidenced upon A-P Lumbosacro-pelvic films, the ovaries are normally found within the boundaries of the lesser pelvis. Films taken after contrast media injections demonstrate that the ovaries are seldom arranged in perfect symmetry. Because these films are taken in the supine position it is not unreasonable to expect a slighty lower position for the ovaries if the imaging examination is conducted in the upright position.

Pathologies, anomalies or other variants may allow the ovaries to rise above the level of the lesser pelvis. Following pregnancy the ovaries usually descend to their normal position within six weeks of childbirth. The ovaries are 8cm-10cm (3"-4") apart in the normal individual, and they are located slightly superior to the transverse axis of the lesser pelvis.

Application of ovarian shielding in daily practice consumes a minimum of time and effort, the benefits of protection certainly outweighing the labor involved. As illustrated, the BCB has a T-shaped velcro-pad band sewn onto its front surface. This T-shaped area allows correct positioning for all male and female gonadal shields.

The shields for A-P views are larger than the ovaries. This allows for a margin of error on two bases:

I. The ovaries may not be positioned symmetrically bilaterally.
II. Even with all due care, placement of the shields may not be perfectly symmetrical.

An imaginary line drawn through both anterior superior iliac spines in the horizontal plane should be 2cm above the superior aspect of the shields. The distance between the shields, center to center, should be 8cm (3"). The vertical axis of the shields should pass medialwards, inferiorly. This ensures that the femoral heads are not obscured. Accurate shield placement will be rewarded by minimal obfuscation of osseous structures. A small portion of the inner ilia and pubes will be shaded, as well as the lateral aspect of the lower sacrum; the coccyx should remain largely visible. (Another quick check to locate the ovaries involves spanning the ASIS and the pubis with one hand, the other hand positioning the shield somewhat medial to the bisected ASIS-pubis line.)

The velcro hook material installed on the posterior surface of each shield needs but slight pressure against the appropriate portion of the BCB's T-strip to be held securely in place. And, as is usual with velcro fastening devices, removal is simply a matter of "peeling" the shield away from the BCB.

A single shield is used for the lateral Lumbosacrococcygeal region examination. It is 9.5cm (3¾") in diameter. Other than its increased size it is constructed exactly the same as the preceding shields.

The shield is placed so that its center is bisected by an imaginary line passing vertically downwards from the anterior border of the body of L4. Viewed on the completed film, the rounded end of the shield should appear adjacent to and nearly fitting into the concave side of the sacrum. No osseous area of interest will be overshadowed if this shield is accurately positioned.

Because these gonadal shields remove almost all of the primary rays the portions of film so protected should, for practical purposes, serve as a base fog test. If shielded areas of completed roentgenographs are dark the shielding may be insufficient, excessive scatter radiation may be present, over-exposure of the patient may have occurred or incorrect film processing may be at fault.

Fig. 8-5 — Testicular shield affixed to BCB in the upright A-P lumbosacral pelvic visualization.

A-Area of Interest
B-Shield in position
C-Placement of shield
D-Resultant Radiograph

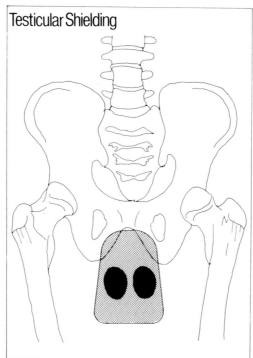

Testicular Shielding

A-Area of Interest

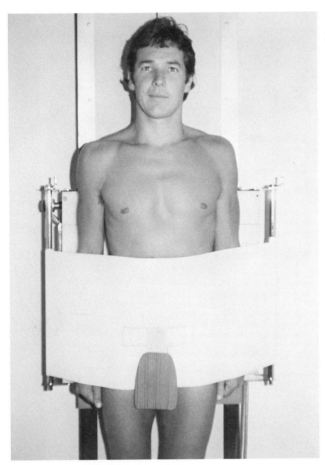

B-Shield in Position

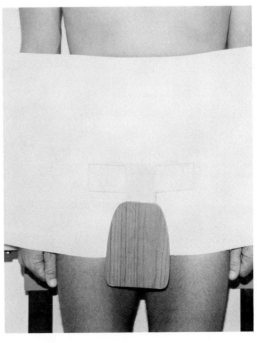

C-Placement of Shield

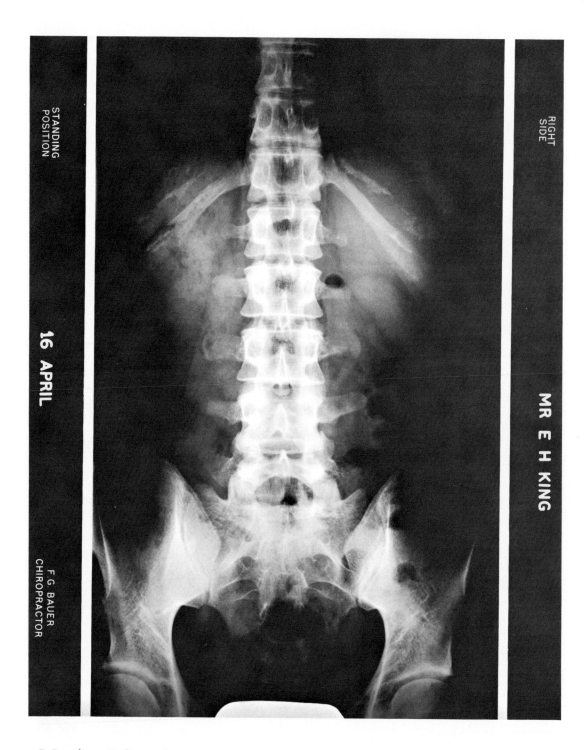

D-Resultant Radiograph

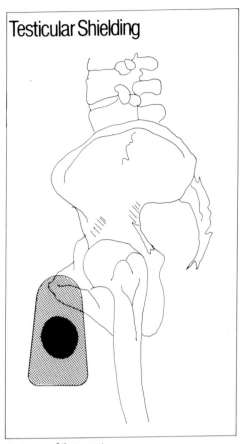

Testicular Shielding

A-Area of Interest

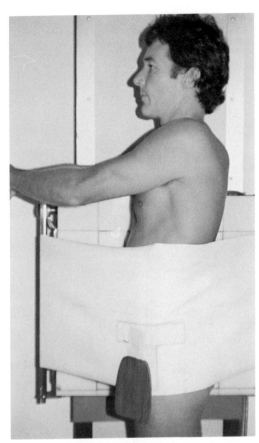

B-Shield in Position on BCB

Fig. 8-6 — Testicular shield affixed to BCB in the upright lateral lumbosacral visualization.

A-Area of interest
B-Shield in position on BCB
C-Placement of shield
D-Resultant radiograph

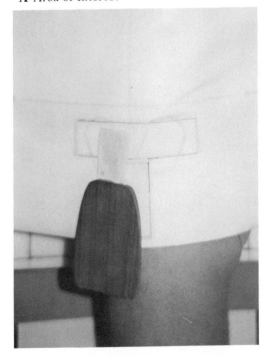

C-Placement of Shield

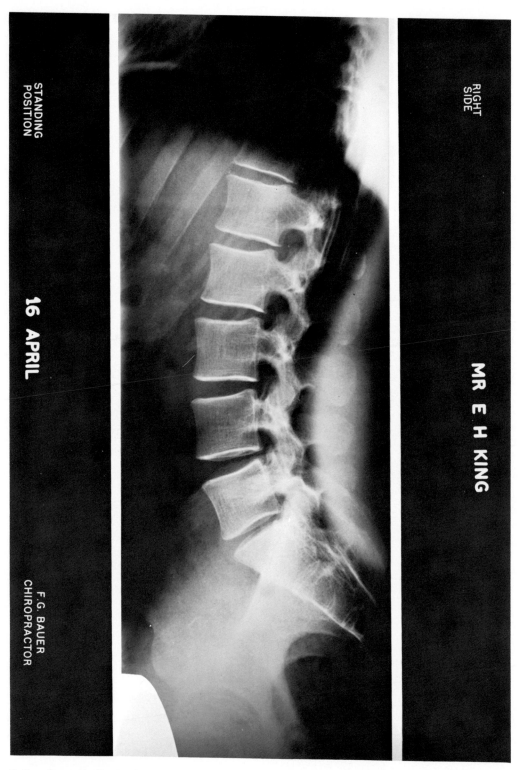

D-Resultant Radiograph

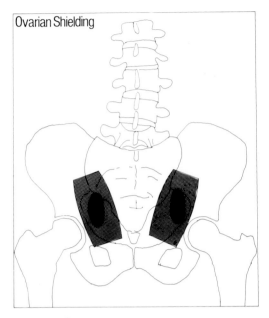

A-Area of Interest

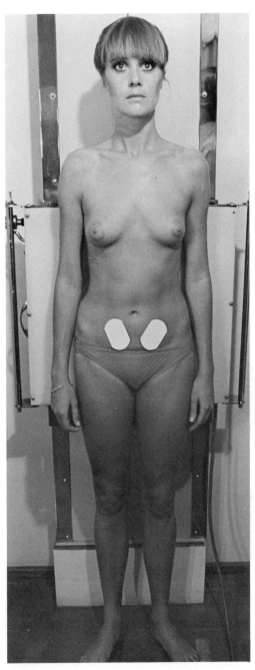

B-Placement of Shields

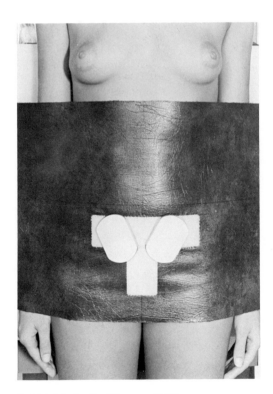

C-Shields in Position on BCB

Fig. 8-7 — Ovarian shields affixed to BCB in the upright A-P lumbosacral pelvic visualization .

A-Area of interest
B-Placement of shields
C-Shields in position on BCB
D-Resultant radiograph

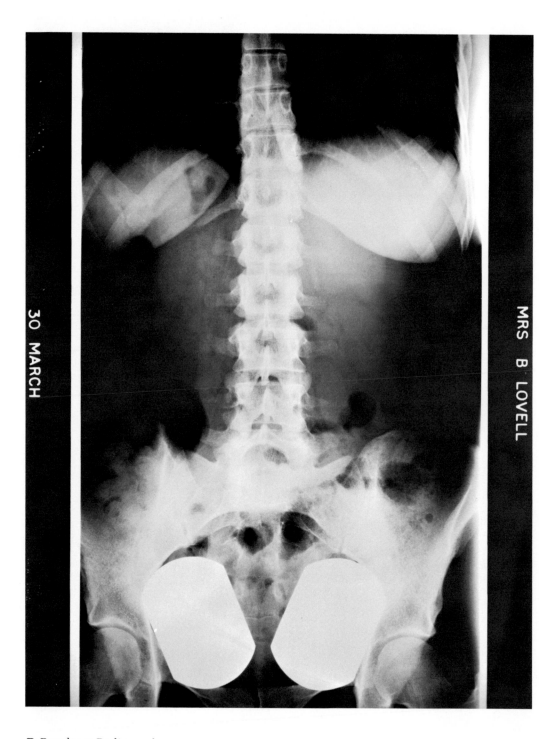

D-Resultant Radiograph

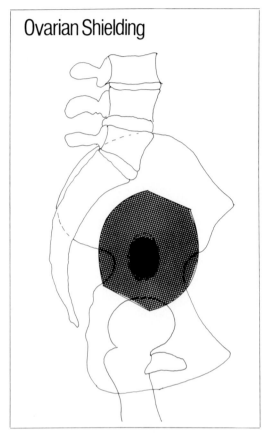

A-Area of Interest

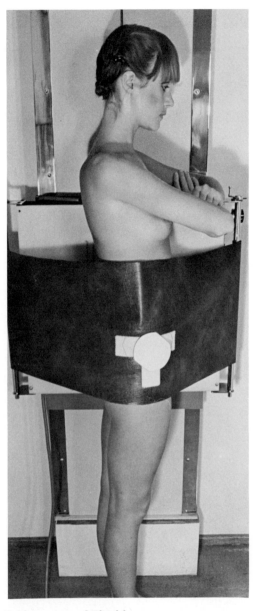

B-Placement of Shield

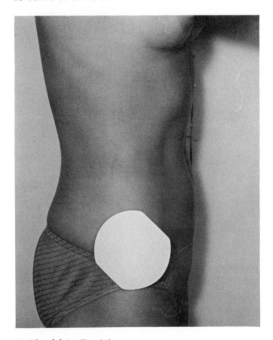

C-Shield in Position

Fig. 8-8 — Ovarian shield affixed to BCB in the upright lateral lumbosacral visualization.

A-Area of interest
B-Placement of shield
C-Shield in position
D-Resultant radiograph

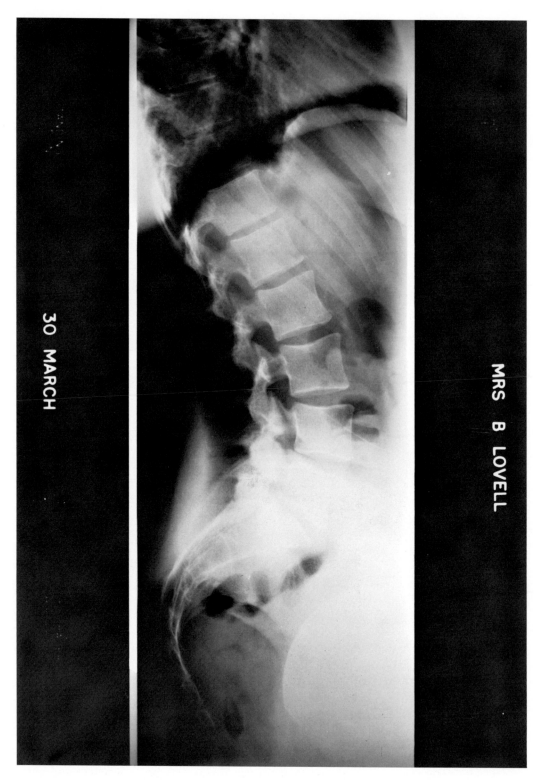

D-Resultant Radiograph

Practical Perspective —

THE EFFECT OF COMPRESSION WITH THE BILATERAL COMPRESSION BAND

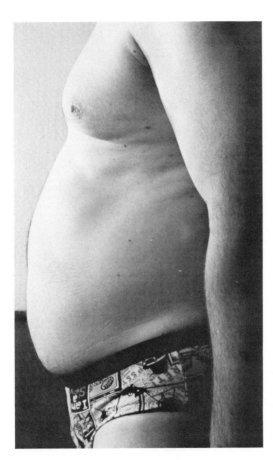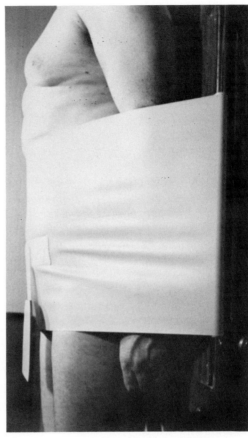

The benefits of compression are readily apparent in the example illustrated above. In the photograph on the left side a middle-aged male is standing upright in a relaxed manner, preparatory to an A-P imaging examination of the lumbar-sacropelvic region. The pendulous abdomen necessitates increased exposure factors for this view and it creates a greater contribution of scatter radiation to the final film result, thus reducing contrast.

In the photograph on the right side, the same patient is seen stabilized with the bilateral compression band (BCB). This procedure effectively eliminates patient movement, improving resolution. Because the thickness of the patient is markedly reduced (from 28cm to 24cm in this instance) there is a decrease in the amount of mAs required to produce the optimum film result. And, a lessened scatter contribution further improves film clarity.

The BCB immobilizes the patient but it does not alter biomechanical considerations. A scoliosis remains unchanged as do any disrelationships existing in the osseous pelvis.

Chapter **9**

Correct Darkroom Procedures

No one has been able to define the physical characteristics of a good quality radiograph in terms useful to everyone, but on the other hand, both the radiology profession and industry agree that a major problem exists in a lack of consistent film processing. Since the advent of automatic film processors, the darkroom has been almost totally ignored, and this poses serious problems in film quality control.

T. T. Thompson, *A Practical Approach to Modern X-ray Equipment*, p. 10, Little, Brown & Co., 1978.

We believe that over 90 percent of poor radiographic results originate in the darkroom, either through processing faults or attendant shortcomings in darkroom design and usage. The reality of these circumstances dictates the approach to this chapter. Practical matters are of utmost importance in the darkroom. Theory provides background knowledge and understanding and is not to be regarded lightly. However, it cannot replace a thorough grounding in the techniques necessary to attain superior radiographic results.

Darkroom design and prerequisites will be dealt with first. Processing procedures and supplemental advice will be reviewed next. Because deeptank hand processing is the method of choice for the highest quality film result it will receive the greatest attention. An explanation of the chemistry involved will follow the pragmatic section and, lastly, guidelines for the use of automatic processing will be considered.

The Darkroom

For convenience of use the darkroom should be situated near the radiographic room whenever possible. It should not be located in either a hot or a damp basement. If the area in which the facilities are located enjoys a warm and sunny climate it is best if the outside wall(s) of the darkroom is/are situated to avoid the hot westerly sun. The air temperature of choice is that of the developer: 20° Celcius or 68° Fahrenheit. Relative humidity is ideally 60 to 65 percent. An ideal entrance is the "maze" method which eliminates the necessity for doors. The disadvantage of this is the floor space required for its effective use. A double-door system provides "insurance" should the outer door be less than light-tight. Another form of darkroom door is the light-proof revolving

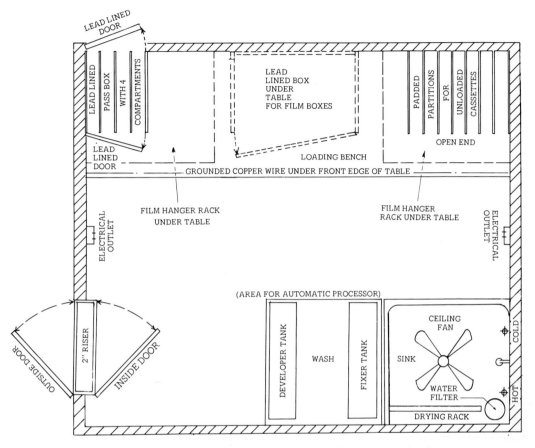

Fig. 9-1 — A well designed darkroom for deep-tank manual processing facilities.

type which operates on the same principle as the revolving doors which used to be popular in department stores. Most x-ray users utilize a single darkroom door; precautions must be taken so that it is thoroughly sealed against the entry of extraneous light from any outside source. A notification system should be installed so that no one enters the darkroom while processing or film handling is taking place. Adequate ventilation is necessary in the relatively confined spaces often encountered in darkrooms; once again care must be taken to ensure light-tight conditions prevail. An example of a well-planned darkroom is illustrated in Fig. 9-1.

Years ago it was thought that walls must be painted black or a dark grey color. Now it is known that light, cheerful colors are more pleasant and, as long as a light-proof status is maintained, quite acceptable in the darkroom. Paint used in the darkroom can be of standard manufacture; a corrosion-resistant variety of oil paint is recommended. Floors should not be slippery nor of a material which stains easily. They should be durable and subject to regular cleaning. Tiles of ceramic or acid-proof rubber types are serviceable, although the former may crack if a solid object is dropped upon them. Certain vinyl tiles are good value and some even provide a degree of cushioning underfoot. Remember to remove spilled solutions at the earliest opportunity; the evaporation of harmful chemicals and their consequent precipitation onto screens or films as dust particles can lead to ultimate film damage.

There is no single perfect size for a deep-tank darkroom although it should be large enough to allow room for easy access to all equipment and supplies. In the normal private practice a room for deep-tank processing should be at least four meters square or, say, seven feet by seven feet in minimal dimensions. If larger floor space is available it can be put to good use. On the other hand, an expansive darkroom is inconvenient, a waste of movement and energy. In the same way that a sink, refrigerator and stove may be awkward to use and require too many steps per job accomplished in a poorly planned kitchen, an ergonomically unsound darkroom places individual film handling and processing tasks too far apart.

Cleanliness is obligatory in the darkroom. If the darkroom is maintained so that it appears to have been installed yesterday, considerable benefit will be derived by its proud owner.

Necessary darkroom equipment is divided into two areas, the *dry side* and the *wet side*. Dry side materials are covered first, with explanatory notes accompanying the various items.

Dry Side

Lead-Lined Film Box. Unless the x-ray room or the darkroom are lead-lined a protective storage cabinet or box is absolutely mandatory to prevent all unexposed film from being affected by ionizing radiation. Even if the x-ray room is lead-lined a container is advantageous to shield films from natural background radiation as well as radiation emitted by materials from which the building is made. A thin layer of lead to arrest scatter radiation in the diagnostic range will suffice for all normal purposes; the recommended measurement is lead 1.5mm thick. Such protection will guarantee freedom from radiation fog for all films while thus stored.

The proper location for the film box is on the dry side, kept off the floor and at a convenient height for the user. It should be constructed so that the sides, bottom, top and door are all leaded, the lead overlapping at each joint. A magnetic catch or suitable latch will keep the door closed when not in use. Vertical partitions to protect film boxes and/or cassettes housed within are useful. Compartments should be large enough to comfortably accommodate the biggest film boxes used. Carpeting on the interior bottom surface will lessen damage to cardboard boxes or cassettes.

If 14" x 36" films are utilized, a lead box of suitable dimensions is of course as necessary as protection for the smaller, more convenient film sizes. Incidentally, the darkroom should be substantially larger to meet the space requirements of the larger films.

Lead-lined loading bins often are used in busy practices and these are quite satisfactory. Non-interleaved film is used in these instances. However, if the x-ray user is prepared to pay the additional cost for interleaved film it will receive added protection from moisture and abrasion.

Loading Bench. The loading bench should be of a large size, ideally running the entire length of the dry wall, and located above the film box. It should be no less than 24" (approximately 60cm) in width and allow for the loading of four cassettes along its length. The surface should be readily cleanable but not hard. A non-static material, such as cork or naugahyde should be affixed to the bench top, constructed so that the front edge is somewhat rounded. No metal trim should be used on the leading edge because it is an invitation to cassette damage. A copper wire secured underneath the entire front edge of the loading bench and going to ground is useful for discharging static electricity from the fingertips.

Film Hangers. There are two types of hangers in common use; the film perforating and non-perforating varieties. The non-perforating hangers grip the film with two opposing, slightly rounded pin points, do not pierce the film itself and are definitely the recommended variety. A slightly underdeveloped small dot near the corners of the film is all the evidence which remains of their use. Film hangers should be cleaned periodically, ensuring that no dried solutions — particularly fixer — remain on the hanger.

Hanger Racks. Brackets for each size of hanger can be mounted either above or below the loading bench. Hangers stored above the bench are more convenient to handle. On the other hand, hangers stored under the bench are located in a safer position because they cannot fall onto cassettes. One incident in which a hanger tumbles upon the interior of an open cassette could very well prove costly.

Cassette Shelves. The best way to ensure that one cassette will not damage another cassette is to make sure that they never come into contact with each other, as mentioned in the last chapter. Vertically partitioned and permanently padded shelves provide individual housing for cassettes while maintaining them in the desired upright position.

Cotton Wool (or cotton balls). This material is very handy for dusting the inside of cassettes when easily removable particles are present.

Shelves for Chemicals. Additional shelving should be installed for storage of developer, fixer and replenisher. If space permits, this shelving should be placed on the wet side of the processing room to reduce the possibility of film and/or screen damage. An ideal location is beneath the sink.

It is advisable to have the ingredients for one complete change of solutions on hand in case supply difficulties arise. Fresh replenisher should always be ready for use, in appropriately sized containers. To keep mixed replenisher in a single, large container allows the remaining contents to become oxidized as replenisher is used. An economical and superior alternative is to put the mixed replenisher in previously emptied small brown beverage bottles, filled to the top and kept well stoppered. As the level of the developer lowers, add the contents of one bottle of replenisher. Remember to stir the solution after adding replenisher.

Towel, Duster, Screen Cleaning Materials. A clean, low-lint towel and duster should be present. Paper towels are not recommended because many brands are laden with lint. Screen cleaning agents which match the requirements of the screens are a necessity.

Pad and Pencil. These items should be within easy reach. The written word is far better for retention of minutiae than the average human mind.

Strong Light. A 100 or 150 watt incandescent light above the loading bench is indispensable. There is no other way to determine if the screens are absolutely clean prior to loading, and screens should be briefly inspected before loading. A fluorescent light should never be used for this purpose because an afterglow will persist for some time after the light is switched off, causing film fog.

Scissors. If a device for rounding corners is not available a pair of scissors is necessary to trim all films, before they leave the darkroom. The spikey, puncture aperture which occurs on films processed with piercing type film hangers readily scratches other films. Scissors are also handy to cut the top off the plastic protective bags found lining film boxes.

Wet Side

There is no singularly unique deep-tank arrangement which is superior to all other types or models. Several varieties are available which will perform quite satisfactorily as long as they are used and maintained properly. An individual tank arrangement can handle the tasks required in a small radiographic installation although an integrated tank system performing as a functional unit is perhaps more advantageous.

Developing Tank. Usually manufactured of stainless steel or a synthetic material, deep-tanks commonly have a capacity of five gallons of solution. They are capable of developing films up to 14" x 17" in size, clipped flat in film hangers. Before putting developer in the tank for the first time, fill the receptacle to the level where the top of the developer should be; only use water for this initial filling. Observe whether the volume of fluid contained is actually five gallons. A discrepancy of + 10 percent may be noted with some tanks, which yields a false developer strength.

Wash Tank. The washing function may be handled by a single tank or by a master tank. The master tank holds developer, fixer and an acid rinse bath tank, if the latter is used. As you face the unit, the developer is to the left, the fixer to the right; wash functions are accomplished in the middle area or compartment. Master tank units usually are made of stainless steel which is a very good material for controlling temperatures of enclosed fluids. Polyvinylchloride (PVC) also is used for tank construction, with the decided advantages of immunity to corrosion and ease of cleaning.

The wash tank may be used as a rinse and a wash tank so the water input and outflow capacities must be ample. A clean, filtered water supply should enter at or near the bottom of the tank and an overflow arrangement be provided to assure a generous water circulation.

Fixer Tank. This tank will be of the same size and material as the developer tank. To avoid spills, splashes and attendant stains an anti-splash panel is a requisite for the front of the tanks. Such a border should extend two to six inches above the top edge of the tanks.

Acid Stop Bath. An acid stop bath aids in prolonging fixer life. It is composed of 98 percent water and two percent acetic acid. Its function is to neutralize the developer remaining upon the film so that development stops immediately. Kept in a separate tank, the acid stop bath should be placed next to the fixer tank.

Dust Cover/Light Lid. All processing tanks should remain covered when not in use, thus excluding dust or other particulate matter. A hinged lid, constructed to be light-tight by virtue of its overlap on the sides of the tank, is a beneficial feature. If necessary, it is possible to leave the darkroom during film processing with the lid in the closed position.

Float & Splash Cover. A light weight inert material is used to make a developer "float." The float rests directly upon the surface of the liquid where it serves to retard oxidation of the developer. Any fixer reaching the developer causes great harm. A splash cover prevents this from occurring in all normal situations. As soon as films have left the developing tank, the float and splash cover should be returned to their usual positions.

Sink. In the darkroom cleanliness is even more important than godliness. A deep sink and a ready supply of hot and cold water are necessary to clean hangers, tanks, various utensils and hands. The clips of film hangers seem to have a natural affinity for residual chemicals. When cleaned occasionally they remain trouble-free. However, the presence of streaks on the completed radiograph informs the x-ray user that hangers require attention.

Stirring Sticks. Various and sundry items have been used to attempt mixing of processing chemicals. Everything from thermometers to eating utensils have been thrown into the fray. Separate stirring sticks are necessary for the developer and fixer, made long enough so that they easily reach the bottom of their respective tanks. A flat piece of plastic or wood which is cut in the shape of a garden spade, the broad bottom section approximately 5" (12cm) long, makes an efficient stirring stick. Label each rod so the fixer stick cannot be inadvertently placed in the developer.

Moving the stirring sticks through a complete circle, as illustrated in Fig. 9-2, ensures complete mixing of a tank's contents and an even distribution of temperature throughout all levels of processing fluids.

The fixer stick should not touch the developer stick and, to lessen chances for error, they should be stored separately. If an immersion heater is used to heat the developer, continue to stir the solution while the heater is operating, thereby promoting an even temperature distribution.

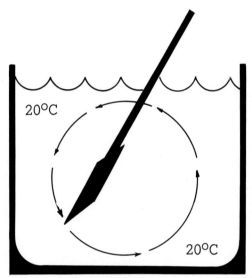

20°C

20°C

RECOMMENDED MOTION
FOR MIXING SOLUTIONS

Fig. 9-2

Thermostatic Controls. It does not matter what the temperature of the developer is just so long as it is either 20° Celsius, 68° Fahrenheit or 20° Centigrade. The only really convenient method of accurately maintaining processing fluid temperature is with a thermostatic control system. Some individuals utilize immersion heaters for warmth and synthetic ice packs for cooling of processing solutions. This is effective but it also is disorderly, messy and unlikely to stimulate much enthusiasm within the involved employee.

Drip Tray. A drip tray is essential to keep water from dropping onto the floor or onto other materials in the darkroom.

Film Hanger Rack. After films have been processed they are installed in a drying rack located above the drip tray. The rack should allow the largest size of film processed to just clear the drip tray. Another lower and separate rack is advisable to keep drops from smaller-sized films from splattering, which will spot the larger films.

Fan or Drying Cabinet. The drying process is considerably hastened with the use of a suitable fan installed above the drying rack. Even better, a thermostatically controlled drying cabinet will achieve complete film dryness within 15 to 20 minutes. Remember to vent a drying cabinet outside the darkroom so that the heat and humidity within will not become elevated.

Thermometer. Even though a thermostatic control system may be installed on the processing tanks, a reliable thermometer serves as a handy reference checkpoint and as a backup in case of a malfunction in the more elaborate system. An installation lacking thermostatic controls requires two thermometers for checking solutions.

Timer. A good quality timer is a very important darkroom implement. One-hour models or luminous watches are not suitable timing devices. The recommended variety is called an *interval timer* and it should be obtained with non-luminous figures for perfect darkroom protection. An interval timer can be used in complete darkness because it has the ability to be pre-set, necessitating only that the operator set it in motion at the appropriate time.

Brush & Sponge. The wash tank should be drained every three to five days, cleaned with a brush, wiped over with a sponge and refilled with fresh water. In busy installations this cleaning routine should be done once a day.

Replenisher. A generous supply should be prepared and stored on "shelves for chemicals," as mentioned earlier in this chapter. If developer becomes weakened, oxidized and/or diluted its reduced strength will require a great increase in milliampereseconds. This results in an elevated radiation dose for the patient, a circumstance to be avoided at all times.

Water Supply. Pure water does not flow from the taps of municipal water supplies. Various substances are found within centralized water systems and many of these impurities are capable of affecting radiographic results. Sand, dirt or rust from pipes may cause tiny white spots to appear on the finished film. Extremely "hard" water may result in precipitation of calcium or magnesium salts, possibly causing white streaks or spots on the film. Sulphides in the water may cause film fogging. If the radiographic installation is located in an area with a problem water supply, distilled water may have to be used for preparation of solutions.

Rural areas that rely upon or augment their water supply with runoff water, held in tanks, will find this a suitable alternative to impure well or bore water. Rainwater, after being held in a storage tank, is several times cleaner than the usual urban water supply. Bore water can be sufficiently purified for radiographic use with the aid of a water filter; a model which operates in the area of 2 -2.5 microns will remove most solids. Commercially distributed "ion exchangers" are effective in demineralizing ion-laden water.

Unless the water supply is satisfactory, tap water is not recommended for use in conventional radiographic solutions. Water that is not good enough to drink is not good enough to use in the preparation of processing solutions.

Viewbox. To allow the earliest possible inspection of processed films a viewbox is necessary in the darkroom. A good location for this built-in illuminator is behind the solution tanks. This facilitates viewing in one area, lessening the hazards of dripping fluids onto the floor or other surfaces from dragging wet hangers around the darkroom.

The viewbox must contain an incandescent light source, not a fluorescent light which could fog unprocessed films. Films must not be viewed until they have been completely "cleared" in the fixer. Also, the fixer and developer must be covered to prevent these solutions from becoming contaminated by runoff from film hangers.

Electrical Outlets. Electrical outlets, called "powerpoints" in British countries, are necessary for thermostatic controls, fans, drying cabinets, etc. Because of the possibility of spillage of water or solutions in the darkroom, all electrical items must be properly earthed as well as precautions taken against the effects of moisture.

"Safelight." There is no such thing as a perfect safelight. An apt descriptive label for a safelight is a *foglight*; safelights can do nothing for the film except fog it. The Agfa-Gevaert organization states this fact (T.D.R./K 12-1-ENG-1975) with exactitude:

> *"Remember that even the best darkroom illumination can cause fogging after a certain time, even on the least sensitive of emulsions. The films should therefore only be exposed to safelight illumination for the time necessary for their handling. Moreover, this handling must be carried out at a sufficient distance from the safelight."*

The use of safelights has probably adversely affected as many films as any other cardinal fault occurring during the handling of x-ray films. That having been said, it is recognized that most x-ray users will continue to use safelights in the darkroom. Therefore, it behooves each individual to adopt prudent habits to lessen the inimical effects of safelight illumination.

Just as films may be developed at any temperature so long as it is 68° Fahrenheit or 20° Celsius, films may be processed in any way as long as it is by the *Time-Temperature Method.* Sight developing with the aid of a safelight is an anachronism to modern radiography. The standardized processing procedures of the time-temperature method allow for the establishment of practices which will guarantee uniformity of results. Further, exposure corrections can be made easily when processing is standardized. The length of time necessary for complete light adaptation, the low level of light within the darkroom, the difficulty of viewing uncleared film and the difference in individual accommodation to greatly reduced illumination are all factors which render sight development inaccurate and obsolete.

Safelights must be of the lowest possible wattage or they will fog films. A 15 watt bulb is more than adequate for general usage. If fast films are being handled a 7½ watt bulb is a necessary precaution against fogging. Safelights should be directed towards the ceiling, ensuring that only indirect illumination reaches the film. If direct safelight illumination is unavoidable the light source should be at least four feet (1.2 meters) from the film.

Various safelight bulbs and filters are available. Be certain that the illumination is correct for the film being used. The simplest method is to obtain a safelight that has provision for interchangeable filters. As an example, x-ray film may be blue-sensitive or green-sensitive. Ensure that your servicing organization has installed the correct filter for the task at hand. Of course, cracked, chipped or otherwise damaged filters do not remain effective.

It is most important to recall that exposed films are far more light sensitive than are unexposed films. As a general guide, exposed films are approximately ten times more sensitive to light than films just removed from the box. This applies especially to films used with intensifying screens. A film that might not be affected by safelight illumination during cassette loading may readily be fogged during cassette unloading and while being installed in a film hanger.

A simple experiment to test possible safelight fogging is done in the following manner:

> Withdraw a fresh, unexposed film from its box in six steps while the safelight is on and the film is in its usual position for cassette loading/unloading. Allow the first area to be exposed for 80 seconds, the second area for 40 seconds, the third area for 20 seconds, the fourth area for 10 seconds and the fifth area also for 10 seconds; the final film section receives no illumination. Now sections of film have been exposed to 160, 80, 40, 20, 10 and 0 seconds of safelight illumination. Develop the film in the usual way. Observe the processed film to determine if various degrees of blackening are present on the film.

If the area of film receiving no illumination shows fogging, remove a film from the box, handle and process in complete darkness and again observe for possible blackening. (If present, the developer may be too warm, the film may be old or it may have been exposed to ionizing radiation or other extraneous light; another inquiry will be necessary to pursue the cause of this problem.)

Repeat the first experiment with a film which has been exposed (preferably with a phantom) using factors which, for example, are typical for an average lateral lumbar examination. Now that a latent image is present on the film, it will be far more sensitive to light from any source. Develop and observe. The number of visibly affected areas discernable on the processed film provides an accurate indication of the effects of a particular safelight.

These experiments must be conducted

with film that is not prefogged in any manner. Another factor to be considered when relating these experiments to the reality of standard processing is time. If several films have been exposed during an examination, loading film hangers one at a time means that the first films installed in the hangers will receive considerably more safelight illumination whenever all films are introduced to the developer simultaneously.

Ancillary Equipment. A plastic bucket is useful to prepare replenisher; this bucket should not be used for any other purpose. The developer stirring stick should be used for this task.

A small plastic funnel assists in filling the small, brown bottles with replenisher. A supply of corks or commercially available metal bottle caps provides stoppers for the replenisher bottles.

Felt or similar soft material is useful to prepare a carrying case for cassettes if they are to be conveyed any distance within the radiographic installation.

Preparing Processing Solutions

Chemicals for developer and fixer are supplied in liquid or powder form, the former being in general usage because of convenience and ease of preparation.

A very brief overview of powder developer usage follows:

Developing powder is supplied in two separate packets. Place contents of one packet into a suitable plastic container, outside the darkroom. This prevents airborne powder from settling upon materials within the darkroom. Mix the powder one spoonful at a time by submerging the spoon's contents into the partially filled developer tank, thus reducing dissemination of the powder into the air. Stir well, then add the contents of the second envelope in the same manner as the first packet. Inadequate, hasty mixing may result in a shortened lifespan for the developer.

Directions for preparing liquid developers are provided by manufacturers.

Before commencing operations make sure that the tanks are quite clean and that no residues of any kind remain within the tanks. Replenisher can be prepared at the same time as the developer; always use replenisher manufactured by the same company that produced the developer.

Mix well with the proper stirring stick. The life of adequately replenished developer theoretically is limitless. However, in practice this is not the case. Colloidal substances are introduced into the developer from the film's emulsion, mechanical impurities may be present, and the sludge which results from this mixture requires regular fluid changes. Once again, when adding replenisher make sure that the "new" solution is well mixed. It is difficult to state a precise figure when discussing the amount of replenisher to add because the amount of aerial oxidation may vary according to conditions. Nevertheless, a practical guide declares that a minimum of 0.4 litres of prepared replenisher should be added for each square meter of film processed.

When dealing with fixing solutions make sure that hardener is added if it is supplied in a separate container. Concentrated liquid fixer has a high specific gravity so if mixing is incomplete only the lower half of films may be fixed. If films appear to be colored with a pink hue in transmitted light and have a green tinge in reflected light, there is too much silver sulphide in the fixer, which is long overdue for a change.

Loading of Cassettes

For optimum results cassettes should be stored in the darkroom in an unloaded state. Films "age" faster if they are not stored in lead-lined boxes; when cassettes are equipped with intensifying screens the enclosed film is even more susceptible to background radiation. Cassettes sometimes are unavoidably kept in conditions of high humidity where moisture can collect within the screens. Then, when films are left in cassettes for a sufficient

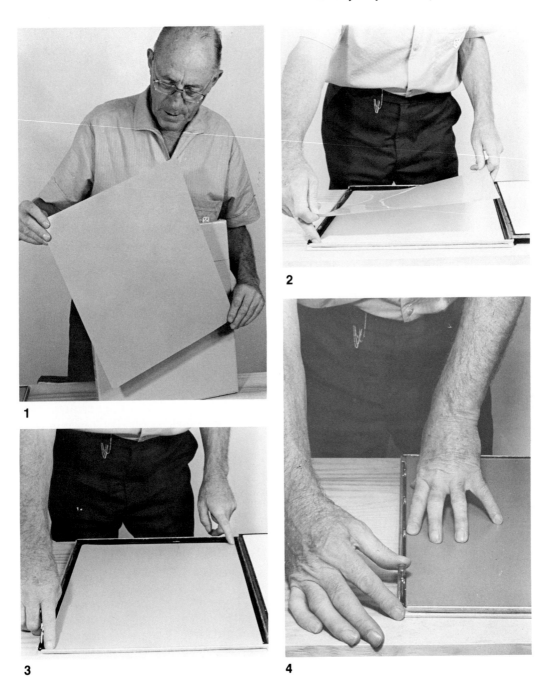

Fig. 9-3 — Care in cassette loading prevents damage to the film.

period of time, over the weekend for example, moisture may leave the screens to be absorbed by the film. These minute amounts of absorbed moisture cause film mottling, generally of a grey, spotty nature, visible on various portions of the processed film.

Preparatory to loading cassettes, switch on a bright incandescent light source over a clean loading bench. Remove cassettes from their storage shelf and place face down on the loading bench, hinges towards and a few inches from the wall. Open cassettes and rest the edges of the back lids against the wall. Inspect the cassettes to see if they are scrupulously clean. Any foreign objects or stains will impair radiographic results so they must be removed before the film is installed in the cassettes. When all cassettes are clean remove the appropriate film box(es) from the lead-lined storage container, place at left on bench, lid upwards. Turn out all lights, including safelight, so that the darkroom is in complete darkness.

Place film box on its narrow side, lid facing operator. Remove lid and place it adjacent to film box. Withdraw films individually from box, ensuring that they are not abraded during handling (Fig. 9-3.1). If interleaving paper is present, remove it from the film and rest it on the bench. Grasp the film between thumbs and forefingers on diagonal corners while placing the little fingers in a downward pointing direction, as illustrated in Fig. 9-3.2. Orient cassette position in the dark with the aid of downward pointing fifth fingers. The horizontally held film is lowered into the cassette, not dragged across the cassette edge. Run a fingertip lightly around the film edge to make certain that the film is positioned properly against the front screen (Fig. 9-3.3). Close cassette back, secure locking devices and proceed with other cassettes in the same manner (Fig. 9-3.4).

After all cassettes are loaded replace each film box lid, turn on overhead white light and replace film box in lead-lined cabinet. The cassettes are now ready for use, with assured confidence that the films have not been prefogged through improper handling. The preceding exhortations may seem unnecessarily pedantic to the reader. That certainly is not the intention. What is strived for is the realization that an accurate "standard operating procedure" must occur if maximum results are to be attained. Circumstances dictate varying conditions in individual installations. Nevertheless, each instal-

lation requires an S.O.P. which will guarantee smooth and trouble-free operations in the darkroom, that most consequential area of radiographic endeavor where a logical, sentient approach to duties is essential.

Film Processing

Upon completion of the patient's radiographic examination, return cassettes to the same position on the loading bench as was used for film loading. Secure the necessary number of appropriate-sized film hangers and lean them against the wall on top of the loading bench, within easy reach of the left hand, so that the top of the hanger is against the bench top or, in other words, upside down.

Open the hinged dust and light cover of the processing solution tank; remove splash covers as well as the developer float. After stirring solutions, check the developer temperature to make sure the thermostat has maintained the temperature at 20° Celsius (68° Fahrenheit). Set the timing clock to exactly four minutes, or to the precise time recommended for the chemistry being used. Discharge any possible static electricity accumulation by touching an earthed copper wire under the front edge of the loading bench; if copper wire is unavailable touching the water taps with fingertips is effective in eliminating static.

Ensure that no extraneous light is entering the darkroom before releasing cassette clasps. (Conscientious practice entails working in total darkness, without safelight.) Stand a cassette on its hinged edge with the cassette front towards the operator. Tilt it back and forth over a short arc. This allows the film to come away from whichever screen it adjoins (Fig. 9-4.1). If the film adheres to either screen, impatience in attempting to scratch it loose with fingernails can only damage the films or the screen. Marks on the screens are permanent and reveal white artifacts on all subsequent films; scratch marks on an individual film

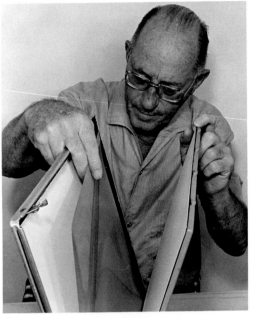

1

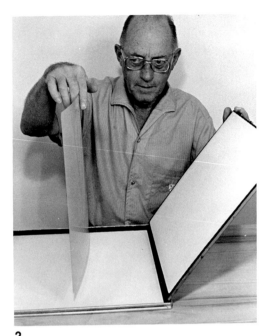

2

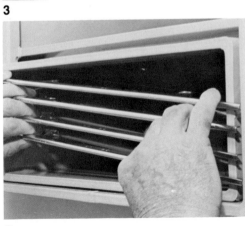

3

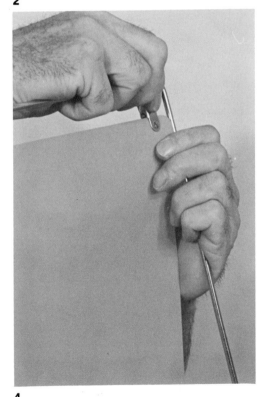

4

5

Fig. 9-4 — The correct method of installing films in hangers. Diagonal insertion of film hangers into processing tanks lessens film scratches and abrasions.

appear dark due to fracture of the emulsion. With a modicum of patience air will soon break the seal which has held the film tightly against the screen.

Once the film is grasped between thumb and forefinger it should be withdrawn vertically to avoid scratching it against the cassette (Fig. 9-4.2). The opposite hand lowers the cassette to the bench top and secures the waiting film hanger (Fig. 9-4.3). The film is installed into the two lower clips first (Fig. 9-4.4), then turned upright for fixing of the top corners. This film should be checked for tautness, particularly along the inferior edge. If loosely joined a flaring film may be scratched by the side of the developing tank.

Repeat the above procedure with remaining films.

To introduce films into the developing tank (four films are the maximum number recommended at one time in a conventional 5 gallon tank), guide them in diagonally over the leading edge of the tank. This method is least likely to allow films to be scratched by the broad vertical side of the tank (Fig. 9-4.5). As soon as hangers are resting on their support shelf activate the preset interval-timer.

Agitation of films should commence immediately and continue for 30 seconds. Agitation removes any air bells which may have formed on the film surface and assists in wetting the film evenly. Another agitation benefit involves a speed-up in the swelling of the film gelatin. The gelatin must swell to allow deep-seated silver bromide crystals to commence development. Without this swelling of the gelatin, final film density and contrast would be reduced. Hangers need only be moved upwards less than ½" (5-10mm) to attain thorough agitation. Repeat agitation for 6 seconds each minute. The movement is best described as an easy shake or jiggle; there is no need to jostle the films about with wild flourishes. Keep hangers apart with the aid of individual fingers used as spacers.

As soon as the timer rings, briskly remove films from the developer and place them in the rinse tank. Do not wait to allow the developing solution to drain back into the tank. The developer which is lodged in and on the film emulsion is spent and is of no further value.

Replace the splash cover on the developer. Agitate films more actively in the rinse compartment. Maintain a good flow of fresh water; the rinse tank should not be a diluted developing tank. After one minute of thorough rinsing remove films and allow to drain for a moment, thus producing minimal dilution of the fixer.

Films also should be agitated in the fixer, to provide quicker and complete fixing. In addition, agitation also prevents film "kissing" and a consequent lack of fixation. The general rule for fixing a film is twice the time necessary to clear it. There is no need to fix a film for 10 minutes if it is clear in 20 seconds. Fresh fixer clears a film quicker than aged, well-used fixer.

Allow processed films to drain back into the fixing tank and then immerse them in fast flowing water for 15 to 20 minutes. Hangers should be well-spaced to allow for the complete removal of all undesirable chemicals. Because of the sulphur content of the fixer, poorly washed films may develop a brownish-yellow discoloration within several months' time.

If an incandescent-lighted viewbox is located behind the solution tanks, the films may be reviewed after a few seconds' washing time. A viewbox so positioned is ideal for early study purposes, preventing the darkroom floor from becoming splotched with stains.

A casual approach to film processing in which an individual pops films into the fixer, waits a few seconds and then turns on the incandescent light source, is risky and unsound. A good habit is to leave the lights switched off until the processed films have entered the wash water.

Once the films have been washed they

should be suspended in a drying rack or placed in a drying cabinet. To reduce the likelihood of water marks occurring on a drying film, loosen the top hanger clips briefly. This aids in dispensing any retained water.

If the film-perforating variety of hanger has been used, the corners of all films should be trimmed when dry, either with scissors or an apparatus designed for this purpose.

While the foregoing does not make inspired reading the material covered does help to make inspired radiographs, and that is what this book is about. To take exceptional quality films, and to preserve minimal radiation dosages for patients, the x-ray user must be ever cognizant of correct darkroom conditions and procedures.

Supplementary Darkroom Advice

Do not add developer when the level of this fluid decreases. The only substance to be used to supplement the developer removed during processing is replenisher. There is a very good reason for this: films being developed liberate bromide. Bromide ions are released from the emulsion as the silver ions are reduced to silver atoms and this bromide remains in the developing solution. The addition of more bromide-bearing developer simply increases the bromide concentration of the solution. Replenisher does not contain bromide and therefore it is the only safe product which can be used to renew the developer. Excessive bromide in the developer produces bromide streaks on films, especially if agitation is conducted inadequately. Bromide streaks are recognizable as darker veins appearing in light areas inferior to dense, dark portions of films. As bromide is liberated during the development process it slowly settles towards the bottom of the tank.

In Chapter V a simple experiment was described wherein "old" film and "new" film was developed and compared to observe the possible presence of fog. A similar experiment with "old" and "new" developer is useful to determine if replenishment has been adequate. The last film processed with the old developing solution and the first film processed with the new solution should have the same density, all other factors being equal. If the film developed in the new solution is darker than the film developed in the old solution replenishment has been insufficient or inaccurate, providing that the first developer has not been allowed to oxidize or otherwise be incorrectly maintained.

The most accurate method for determining replenishment requirements is to maintain a record of all films developed and the size of each film. Because this may prove overly burdensome, it is sufficient to remove films briskly from the developer, allow no run-off into the developing tank, and simply add replenisher as required. A dependable guide provides for the addition of 400 cubic centimeters of replenisher for every square meter of film developed, or approximately 12 ounces of replenisher for 11 square feet of film developed.

How often does the x-ray user change developer? If a 5 gallon tank is being employed and the manual processing facility is not consistently busy, fresh developer should be prepared for every 150 films processed or once each month, whichever occurs first. Before scoffing at this seemingly short interval remember that the cost of developer is moderate and the amount of work accomplished by the developer is exceptional. The x-ray photons are responsible for the formation of a latent image; then the developer magnifies this latent image by a factor of 10,000,000 and more, demonstrating the importance of accurate processing with full-strength solutions.

Fixer need not be changed more often than every three months if the same criteria are applied to fixer as were applied to developer in the preceeding paragraph. Fixer weakens by dilution, not by oxidation. Films will require an increased time period for clearing and hardening as fixer ages; however, this is not as unequivocably critical as the developer status and so an increased time-frame is acceptable.

All cassettes should be clearly identified with a broad-tipped marking pen. The top end of each cassette should be labeled to facilitate proper placement in the bucky tray and for ready reference when installing films in hangers preparatory to processing. Processed films can then be readily viewed in the normal upright position while wet. Viewing wet films in a hanger turned upsidedown may lead to streaks appearing on dried films along a vertical line corresponding to the location of the superior film clips. If a manufacturer's label giving screen identification is not present this information should also be placed on the cassette front.

There is a fallacy currently being promulgated in some quarters which declares that a properly exposed film is impossible to overdevelop. Like many other statements this one contains elements of truth which have resulted in an erroneous conclusion. Of course it is possible to overdevelop a film. The premise behind the impossible-to-overdevelop hypothesis is that only those portions of the film subject to exposure are develop-able, and this assumption may appear to be accurate from a theoretical basis. Nevertheless, from practical experimentation any x-ray user can confirm the fact that fog increases if films are markedly overdeveloped. After a while film crystals that were not subject to exposure begin to be developed. Now this development fog will not make the black areas appear to be any blacker but it will certainly cause the white areas to become more grey, decreasing contrast and decreasing the average gradient of the film. Even though blacks do not become blacker an overall increase in density certainly affects image quality.

Most assuredly x-ray film can be over-developed.

The *clearing* of a film being fixed refers to the fading of the "original milky opaqueness" which is still present after developing and rinsing have been completed. The fixer removes undeveloped silver halide during the clearing period.

To determine the clearing time of fresh fixer use a small flashlight to check upon the progress of an experimental film in the fixing tank. (The last time the authors conducted this test the first film was cleared in less than 20 seconds, prior to the first inspection. The second film was observed from 10 seconds onwards, becoming completely "clear" in an abrupt manner between 13 and 15 seconds following immersion.) With the aid of a flashlight inspect the test film every few seconds; ascertain and make note of the time taken for the film to become completely clear. Repeat this procedure with a test film after several weeks' use of the fixer. In normal circumstances a considerable length of time is required to clear films with old fixer as compared to new fixer. Note the clearing time for both new and old fixer to eliminate future fixing-time guesswork.

Never grasp a film with fingernails even if the film is inside the folded interleaving paper. Film emulsions are easily fractured, allowing overdevelopment to occur at the site of fracture. Do not allow a sharp edge or corner of a film to contact a screen because the sensitive screen surface is readily susceptible to damage. Do not use fingers in an attempt to remove foreign matter from a wet film; a piece of cotton-wool is suitable for removing particulate objects which may be adhering to the wet film surface.

Do not attempt to correct exposure errors by underdeveloping. Only when films are being correctly processed by accurate and standardized processing methods can one contemplate working out an appropriate exposure technique, with a particular x-ray machine, in a particular locality with a particular electrical line supply, taking into account variations in film and screen speeds, grid ratio, tube target wear, object size and density variations. It takes diligent application to become a radiographic imaging virtuoso; the best place to begin this edification is within the darkroom.

Darkroom Chemisty

Development is the process which renders a latent image visible. As with conventional photographic developer, radiographic developer is a chemical reducing agent converting silver ions into silver atoms. Film crystals that are struck by photons during the imaging examination become ionized. Chemical processing of the film reduces the ions to atoms, thereby resulting in black silver being deposited at film sites where exposure has taken place. Where exposure has not taken place no ionization occurs, no development occurs and these areas become relatively transparent following fixation.

For silver halide crystals, development is an all-or-none reaction. If a sensitivity speck is activated within a crystal during latent image formation, that speck permits development to proceed. If no radiation reaches the crystal, no development occurs (modifying factors aside). The prevailing grey areas which appear on the completed radiograph are the result of ionization of incomplete numbers of crystals during exposure, not incomplete development of individual crystals.

Two developing agents usually are found in the developing solution. Hydroquinone is used in conjunction with metol or phenidone depending on the manufacturer concerned. Two developing agents are used because the combination produces development which is faster and more thorough than that occurring with the use of single agents; this phenomenon of improved developer reaction is termed *synergism* or *superadditivity*.

In addition to the developing agents, the developer contains activators, preservatives and restrainers.

An *activator* is needed because developers will only function properly in an alkaline medium. In addition, the alkali aids in controlling the hydrogen ions which become available through the development process. Common activators include sodium carbonate, potassium carbonate, sodium hydroxide and borates.

Oxygen in the air will readily oxidize an alkaline developer, rapidly lessening its effectiveness. A *preservative* is necessary to render the colored endproducts of development harmless, and to reduce oxidation. Sodium sulfite is the most commonly used preservative.

Development of unexposed crystals results in the formation of *chemical fog*; its appearance is heralded by a uniform, grey cast to the film. A *restrainer*, or *antifoggant*, is necessary to prevent the developing agents (especially phenidone) from uncontrolled activity. Potassium bromide is the prevalent restrainer in current radiographic usage. Minute amounts of lesser additives often are utilized by manufacturers of developers; there is no need for a review of these substances in this treatise.

The requirements of a fixing bath call for clearing of the film, followed by its hardening for permanent safekeeping. In order to clear the film a substance is needed which will remove the unexposed silver halide crystals. (If undeveloped silver halide crystals are allowed to remain on a poorly fixed film the silver will discolor with age and/or exposure to light, yielding that familiar, brown-tarnished appearance.)

Thiosulfate is the compound capable of this task, applied in the form of ammonium thiosulfate or sodium thiosulfate. The latter compound is called "hypo" and it has been used by photographers for decades.

In addition to the "hypo" (functioning

as a remover of silver halides from the emulsion) several fixation additives are utilized. Weak acids neutralize any alkaline developer transported to the fixing tank. Sodium sulfite again is called upon to act as a preservative of fixer as well as of developer. Finally, a *hardener* is added. Potassium alum or a chromium or an aluminum compound are the standard hardening reagents. A hardener lessens swelling of the gelatin, keeps it from softening in the wash water and improves its abrasion resistance.

Automatic Processing

In recent years more and more x-ray users have been rejecting hand processing methods and turning to automatic processing systems. In an age of automation this is quite understandable. Still, anyone contemplating the purchase of automatic processing equipment should give the matter careful thought prior to its acquisition, not several months after the machinery is installed.

Automatic processing concerns the same basic chemistry as that involved in hand processing; it is simply a procedure utilizing more aggressive chemicals at higher temperatures. Just as a commercial film lab cannot compete with the results obained by hand processing in the darkroom of an avid photographer, automatic processing in radiography is generally inferior in quality to manual film treatment. Optimal automatic processing simply does not equal optimal manual processing.

If the installation routinely handles less than 40 films per day automatic processing is ill-advised. Prospective purchasers sometimes are unaware of the scrupulous care needed to keep automatic processing equipment in faultless condition. Their mind's eye may simply see a film being inserted in a slot and a completed roentgenogram appearing as if by magic. If servicing requisites are not carried out by the operator, comparatively costly maintenance duties must be attended to by an outside firm, else imaging results will fall short of ideal.

Automatic processing certainly does enable a greater volume of films to be expedited, freeing hands and minds for other tasks. And, the degree of standardization that occurs with its use could be of great benefit to x-ray facilities obtaining uneven results. All films are developed exactly alike in automatic processing. There is no "pulling" of films after two minutes if they seem to be "overdone," as may be carried out with sight development. Any deficiencies in exposure techniques must be remedied at their source, a beneficial side-effect of automatic processing.

Mr. K. R. Jackson, F.I.R., Technical Specialist with the Dupont organization, has authored the following contribution on practical aspects of automatic processing:

Practical Aspects of Automatic Processing

With ever increasing demands on x-ray facilities, automatic processing is vital to obtain diagnostic radiographs in the shortest possible time.

It often is stated that a film processed manually is superior to a film processed automatically, but this need not be so if strict guidelines are observed.

There are many factors to consider if one is contemplating the purchase of an automatic processor. An abbreviated review of these factors follows, classified into ten areas of interest.

1. Choice of Equipment

If less than 100 films per day are to be processed, a low capacity unit should be considered, one with an increased dwell time of at least 25 seconds in developer and fixer.

"Time saving" has to be the main reason to purchase an automatic processor for less than 40 films per day. There are many pitfalls in automatic processing and a potential user must be committed to a high daily replenishment rate and a change of chemistry at no less than two-week intervals.

2. Processing Area

The space required for an automatic processor need only be large enough to accommodate the processor, replenishment tanks (2), sink (large enough to wash the film transport racks), a film hopper and a loading bench. The processor can be fully or partially enclosed in a darkroom, or it can be free-standing for daylight application.

If the processor is to be kept in a darkroom, the room must be completely light tight and possess ample ventilation. The services needed are electricity, water and drainage. If film is to be stored in the darkroom, ideally the temperature should be 70°F with a relative humidity of 40-60 percent. Chemistry should never be stored near film.

3. Processor Systems

There are six main systems:

(i) Transport
(ii) Electrical
(iii) Replenishment
(iv) Recirculation
(v) Water
(vi) Dryer

All these systems must be checked regularly and specifications suggested by the manufacturer must be adhered to strictly.

4. Chemistry

Because of the close tolerances needed in automatic processing due to higher temperatures and shorter dwell times, special additives have to be used to allow the film to swell and harden rapidly during transportation through the roller system.

The basic ingredients are much the same as for manual processing, the main difference being the inclusion of hardeners such as Gluteraldehyde for the developer and Aluminum Chloride or Postassium for the fixer.

As the developer is hyper-active when first mixed, a starter solution must be used to bring the working solution to a normal level and to create a balanced mixture. Usually 23.5cc's per liter are added to new chemistry in the processor, not in the replenishment tank.

5. Special Considerations When Mixing Chemistry

(a) Solutions are to be mixed according to the manufacturer's instructions.

(b) Keep replenishment tanks clean — oxidized chemistry must be cleared off the sides before a remix is initiated.

(c) Check replenisher tank volumes regularly — they can become distorted after regular mixing.

(d) Use a different mixing paddle for the developer and the fixer and always wash each paddle thoroughly.

(e) Use a clean, non-absorbent material for a floating lid for the developer replenisher tank; this step markedly reduces oxidation of the solution.

(f) Always wear safety glasses.

6. Optimum Processing Standards

To obtain optimum results with any processing system, it is imperative that a Quality Control Program be implemented to monitor any variation or changes that may occur. It is, therefore, of great value that some knowledge be gained of film sensitivity and the common causes of unsatisfactory radiographs. As in manual processing, the automatic system is controlled by the same three parameters: time, temperature and activity. It is possible to use a combination of any of these three, but the controlling factor is the time the film remains in the developer tank. This obviously is controlled by the speed of the processor. Time is critical — a two or three second change can make a difference to the final radiographic result. With a stopwatch the dwell time of the film is recorded. This means that timing commences when the leading edge of the film enters the chemistry and ends when the leading edge exits the chemistry. The known dwell time in combination with knowledge of the chemistry activity will then influence the temperature.

7. Replishment Rates

To obtain the correct replenishment rates of chemicals an average of film usage has to be estimated, either by number of films processed or, preferably, by square footage. There are many formulae that can be used, but satisfactory results can be gained by using as a basis the folowing:

Under 100 films (mixed sizes) per day:
Developer - 80cc's per 14" travel of film
Fixer - 180cc's per 14 " travel of film

Over 100 films (mixed sizes) per day:
Developer - 65cc's per 14" travel of film
Fixer - 100cc's per 14" travel of film

8. Monitoring of Processor

It is not necessary to purchase expensive equipment to carry out test procedures for processor performance. It must be remembered, however, that whatever device or film strips are being used have to be checked regularly against a known standard prepared when all conditions are known to be exact. A device called a sensitometer, which enables a known density range to be exposed on a double or single emulsion film is ideal although expensive. The exposed film is then processed and the various densities either read by a densitometer or compared visually. If pre-exposed density wedges are used by your service personnel, it is important to be aware of latent image regression and possible increase in base fog due to aging.

Because all x-ray departments have exposure equipment, perhaps the easiest way to monitor processor performance is with the aid of an aluminum step wedge. This method is accurate only if the following conditions are adhered to:

(a)   The x-ray unit is in peak condition.

(b)   The same factors are always used.

(c)   The same cassette and screens are used.

(d)   Film is taken from the same box, which has been stored in a cool area.

(e)   The same collimation is used.

9. Maintenance

A processor is very much like a motor car; unless it is properly looked after it will not perform well. It is important, therefore, to set up a maintenance program for any automatic processor. Suggested daily and weekly procedures are as follows.

Daily:

(i)   Check temperature with an outside thermometer.

(ii)   Remove and clean top crossovers.

(iii)   Wipe top of rollers with a clean, warm sponge (to remove oxidized and crystalized chemistry). N.B. Never use the same sponge for the developer and fixer.

(iv)   Check water supply — a good flow is important.

(v)   Check recirculation of chemistry.

Weekly:

(i)   Remove one rack per week and check all cogs and springs.

(ii)   Place rack in a sink which is large enough to allow complete immersion and

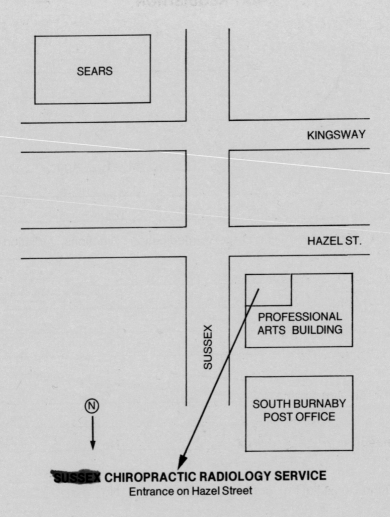

SUSSEX CHIROPRACTIC RADIOLOGY SERVICE
Entrance on Hazel Street

SID E. SHE   C C.R.
Doctor of Chiropractic
I 4 - 6035 SUSSEX STREET
BURNABY, B.C. V5H 3C1
PH: 438-6106

X-RAY REQUISITION

Dr. FOLLIS

5203 VICTORIA DRIVE

PT. Name __BROWN.__ M__ F__ Age 29

Address / 5531 FOREST. ST.

BBY __ Tel.__

HISTORY (fractures, major surgery, medication, injections, radiation therapy)

— treated by DC – 3Y – then unremitting Sciatica on wkend.

Study Requested-Spine: AP, LAT.

Extremity: __

Written report   Yes __ No__

Telephone Consultation   Yes __ No ▬▬

ICBC (Claim # /Centre) __

WCB (Claim #) __

Private Exam __

Patient Pick Up X-Rays   Yes __ No__

clean thoroughly. Use a
sponge and nylon brush
but never add detergent.

A special systems cleaner is necessary
every three months for the developer
rack.
N.B. Never splash fixer into the developer.
This contaminates the developer.

Preventive Maintenance:
It can be very expensive and time consuming if an unscheduled breakdown
occurs. It is wise, therefore, to plan a
scheduled maintenance program with the
manufacturer's representatives, who will
provide you with servicing guidelines.

10. Problem Solving
   A discussion of the following possible
problem areas may provide assistance to
the x-ray user experiencing various film
artifact irregularities:
   (A)   Film Fogging
   (B)   Mechanical Impediments
   (C)   Film Contamination
   (D)   Manufacturing Faults
   (E)   Electrical Discharge

(A) Film Fogging (Increase in Base
   Fog):
   Artificial Light — The safelight
      may be too close to the
      workbench; it may have a bulb
      of incorrect wattage or the
      safelight filter may be worn or
      fractured.
   Daylight — Daylight may enter
      through cracks around doors or
      windows, or around cassette
      margins from damage to clasps,
      or light may even enter faulty
      film storage bins.
   X-ray Irradiation — Fogging may
      be due to x-ray beam effects
      upon unshielded darkroom
      walls, cassettes or film storage
      bins.
   Backscatter caused by photons
      energizing material placed
      within the range of cassettes
      may increase fog levels.

Age — Outdated, deteriorated film
   and chemistry can result in
   increased fogging effects.
Chemistry — Hyperactive
   developer, elevated temperature
   of processing solutions and
   contamination of developer and
   fixer may yield increased fog.
Lack of patient compression,
   improper grid ratio or
   inadequate collimation may
   individually or severally
   increase film fogging.

(B) Mechanical Impediments:
   Kink Marks (black and white) —
      These artifacts may be caused
      by improper handling and/or
      storage conditions.
   Scratches — Scratches can result
      from careless film loading and
      unloading procedures; from dirt
      on workbenches, screens and
      processor trays; from faulty
      crossovers and rollers, or from
      dirty crossovers and rollers.

(C) Film Contamination:
   The surface of the film may be
      contaminated by
      - the splashing of chemistry or
      water;
      - grease and perspiration from
      hands;
      - drying marks caused by
      inadequate washing and drying
      procedures.

(D) Manufacturing Faults:
   Artifacts can result from
      "emulsion misses"; fine line
      streaks and abnormal drying
      patterns may occur as a result of
      faults encountered during the
      film manufacturing process.

(E) Electrical Discharges:
   Static discharge (originating from
      friction, pressure or adhesion
      defects) may be caused by
      - low natural humidity or non-
      humidified air conditioning;

- lack of earthing of loading benches;

- flooring material and clothing, nylon being the worst offender.

Chapter **10**

Film Presentation

Efficient utilization and maximum extraction of information carried by the x-ray image is one of the most challenging problems currently faced by radiologists.

R. J. Schulz, *Diagnostic X-ray Physics,* p. 55, GAF Corporation, 1977.

Film Viewing

The subject matter for consideration in this chapter is not overly long. Nevertheless, it is quite important. For what shall it profit a man if he shall gain a superior quality film and lose his diagnosis due to poor viewing conditions?

The prevailing method of examination during roentgenology's formative years was fluoroscopy, not radiography. Advances in film and equipment occurred more rapidly in the latter mode and resulted in the adoption of conventional roentgenology as the standard in everyday practice. There are noteworthy differences between viewing a fluoroscopic screen and viewing a properly processed x-ray film.

Physiology of Vision

Under conditions of normal illumination the eye sees with cones. When light levels fall the other visual receptors, rods, become active. Cones are located mainly in the fovea where rods are entirely absent. Rods predominate throughout the remainder of the eye, being in greatest concentration approximately 20 degrees from the fovea. Because rods are absent from the central viewing area of the eye the fluoroscopic viewer does not concentrate directly on the image. Instead, he will look around the normal line of vision and he will keep his eyes in fairly continual motion, for rod vision is more acute with moving than with stationary objects.

When the light level drops, the rods are not immediately effective. These receptors take from 30 minutes to one hour to attain their maximum perception of contrast. That is why it is unwise to make a visual inspection of any darkroom shortly after entering the area. At least 15 minutes must pass before satisfactory dark adaptation takes place.

So it is with the intending fluoroscopist. He must wait 15 to 20 minutes for adaptation to occur. As rods do not react to red light, wearing red goggles allows him to dark adapt before proceeding with the examination. The resultant red-cone vision is acute enough to allow for the

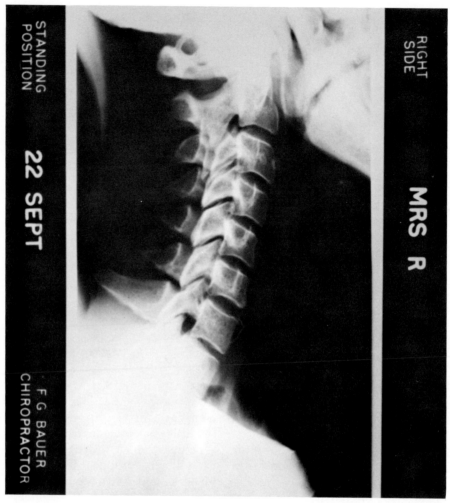

STANDING POSITION

22 SEPT

F G BAUER CHIROPRACTOR

RIGHT SIDE

MRS R

Fig. 10-1 — Viewing A Film: **A**
"A" — with surrounding extraneous light

conduct of everyday activity prior to the fluoroscopy exam.

Of course, the advent of image intensifiers has changed the rules of the earlier game. Dark adaptation no longer is required with modern image intensifiers which magnify brightness between 5,000 and 10,000 times.

Rod vision is far less acute than is cone vision. The term *visual acuity* describes the sharpness that is present in different forms of sight. This quality is measured by numbers of line pairs. A line pair is one line and one space, the space being the same width as the line; the unit of measurement is a millimeter. During optimal performance of cone vision the eye will resolve 1.5 to 2 line pairs per millimeter over a span of 20 centimeters. During the reduced capabilities of rod vision 0.2 line pairs per millimeter are visible, demonstrating the vast superiority of detail perceptible to cone-lit circumstances.

The final comparison in vision physiology pertaining to fluoroscopy-radiography concerns integration time. This is the time period over which the eye is

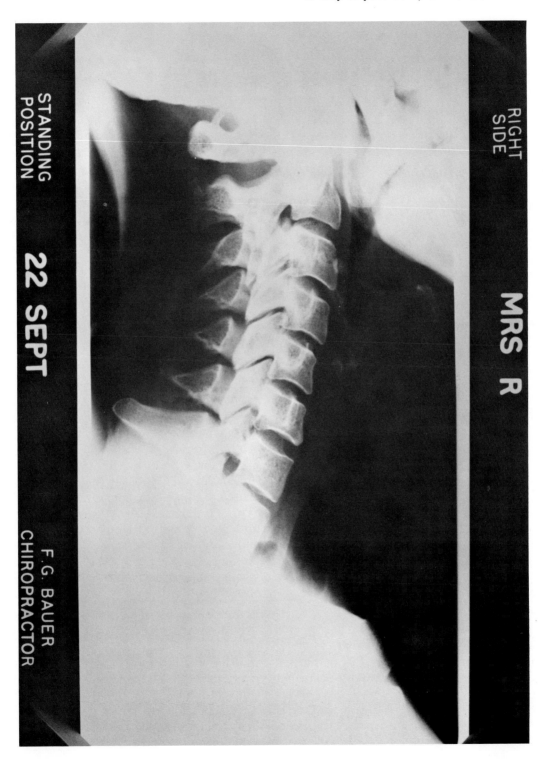

Fig. 10-1—"B"— Without surrounding extraneous light.

capable of forming, or accumulating or integrating image information. The human eye can only store information for 0.2 seconds after which time a new picture must be created. The x-ray film stores information in perpetuity, exempt from the limits of the eye. Staring at an image on a fluoroscopic screen for lengthy intervals does not benefit the viewer with an improved image. Of course, film provides a higher quality image than fluoroscopy, simply from the number of photons affected in a radiographic exposure.

Viewing X-ray Films

A processed film can be reviewed to best advantage when mounted upon a quality viewbox set in favorable conditions. The human eye sees best at a certain level of illumination. Thankfully the pupillary light reflex makes corrections when there is too much or too little light impinging upon the retina. Figure 10-1 illustrates the relevance of this fact to radiology.

The film 10-1 (A) occupies the entire area of illumination while the film 10-1 (B) is surrounded by light. (A) is much easier to read than (B) and more liable to offer up an accurate impression of the examined area. In (A) the pupil is dilated in comparison to (B) yielding maximum contrast and perception. The extraneous light in (B) causes the pupil to constrict, lessening the amount of light perceived through the x-ray film.

Viewboxes

The viewbox should provide a strong white light as a source of illumination. Light sources of different hues are not recommended because they will influence the vision of the film reviewer when he is visiting other facilities where standard lighting is present.

The source of illumination should be fluorescent lighting, not incandescent lighting. The latter tends to create uneven light patterns and also generates a great deal of heat. The fluorescent tube must be of adequate strength to completely illuminate the viewing surface. The light source must be placed deep enough in the viewbox to allow direct and reflected light rays to create even illumination. A translucent type of glass ("flashed opal" glass is a recommended variety) is more suitable for the viewing surface than a plastic material. Plastic derivatives scratch more easily than does glass and a constant impediment to the film image may result. The translucent surface of the glass should be against the film for correct viewing.

The entire inner surface of a viewbox must be kept clean if maximum reflection and visibility are to be maintained. Naturally the exterior viewing surface must also be spotless. Mirrors or other reflecting media may be added to the inside of a viewbox to improve its performance.

The best viewboxes have variable intensity lighting which aids in lessening the shortcomings of radiographs incorrectly exposed or processed. "Spot lights" are available which provide intense illumination for small areas in those instances where a film is darkened due to overexposure. All the viewboxes in a particular facility should be of a comparable and satisfactory standard. It would be shameful to order retake films on a patient, only to discover that the viewbox was at fault.

Ambient light in a film reading room should be maintained at a reduced, nondistracting level. High levels of room lighting can cause reflections from the film surface leading to degradation of image quality. Because visual acuity differs among individuals it is necessary to consider all aspects of film viewing so that optimal conditions can be maintained. Also, optical preferences exist among film reviewers, a fact which prevents complete standardization within the x-ray world.

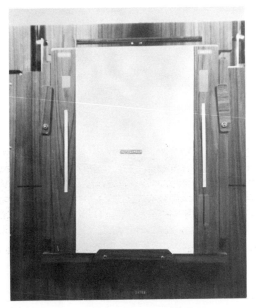

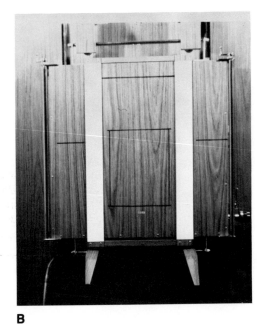

A   **B**

Fig. 10-2 — Lead masks used for 14″ x 17″ film:
"A" — when applying film identification
"B" — when making the patient exposure

Patient Preparation

The simplest and most effortless way of conducting an x-ray examination of torso areas is to have the patient completely unclothed. Since western society maintains a degree of modesty precluding such an examination, the next best thing should be done. The patient should be gowned if female, reduced to undershorts if male.

Obviously, the gown should not have zippers or buttons. Depending on the area(s) being examined, various items must be removed. Hair pins, glasses, earrings and jewelry are nothing more than potential artifact creators. Dentures fit the same category. Shoes may create biomechanical distortion in the person being examined. Bra fasteners do nothing to enhance film results; underwired bras are even worse. In general, clothing is detrimental to film quality. The well known "end on" effect of even lightweight material can be distracting to the film viewer and image degradation is always a possibility.

Film Identification

The usual method of film identification utilizes a small typed form whereby the information content is transferred to the x-ray film via a photoprinter. This method is an adequate form of identification and it enjoys widespread use.

The F. G. Bauer-produced films appearing in this book are labeled with lead letters affixed to the bucky front. Their appearance is remarkably crisp because the film margins were exposed at 40 kVp instead of the 100 kVp used for the body-part images. Connoisseurs of the x-ray plate as an art form may wish to emulate these methods.

Fig. 10-2 shows the bucky-mounted overlays which are used to produce the distinctive appearance of the films in this text. When the required number of films necessary for a patient examination has been determined, shields of 1.5mm lead thickness are placed in position over that part of the film which will constitute the patient occupied area of imaging interest. For example, the usual lateral lumbar

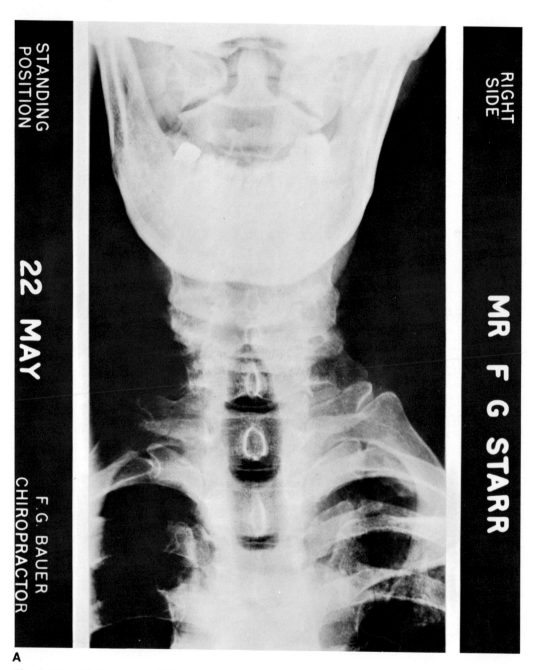

STANDING POSITION

22 MAY

F.G. BAUER CHIROPRACTOR

RIGHT SIDE

MR F G STARR

A

Fig. 10-3 — Well presented films of the cervical ("A" & "B") and lumbosacral ("C" & "D") regions. Note the upper thoracic segments included in the A-P cervical view and the even exposure of segments from coccyx to T10 in the lateral lumbar view.

view can be placed on 15cm (6") of film. This central film area is shielded by the lead overlay, the necessary data is applied to the bucky front, and an exposure of 40 kVp and 32 mAs for fast screens or 64 mAs for high-definition screens "prints" the information onto the film. After each film has been data-printed the patient is exposed using the appropriate cassette for each view. A lead shield covers the

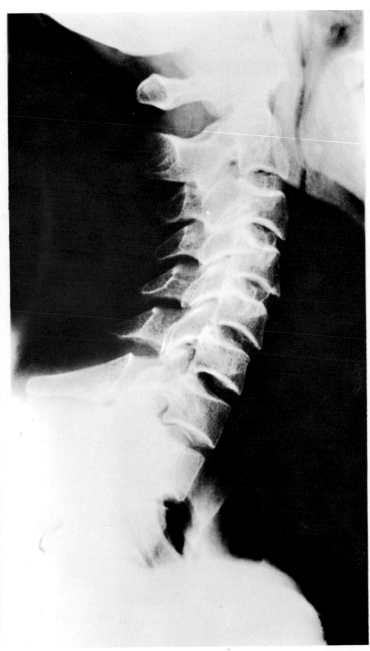

STANDING POSITION   22 MAY   F.G. BAUER CHIROPRACTOR

RIGHT SIDE   MR F G STARR

B

already labeled portion of the film so that scatter is prevented from causing degradation of the recorded images.

It is true to say that the collimator could be left with shutters opened wider than necessary and the lead overlay would prevent this from being noticeable.

However, it is logical to assume that one who has paid so much attention to all other aspects of quality film presentation would not become careless with collimation.

Aside from the obvious aesthetic benefits in producing such an attractive film,

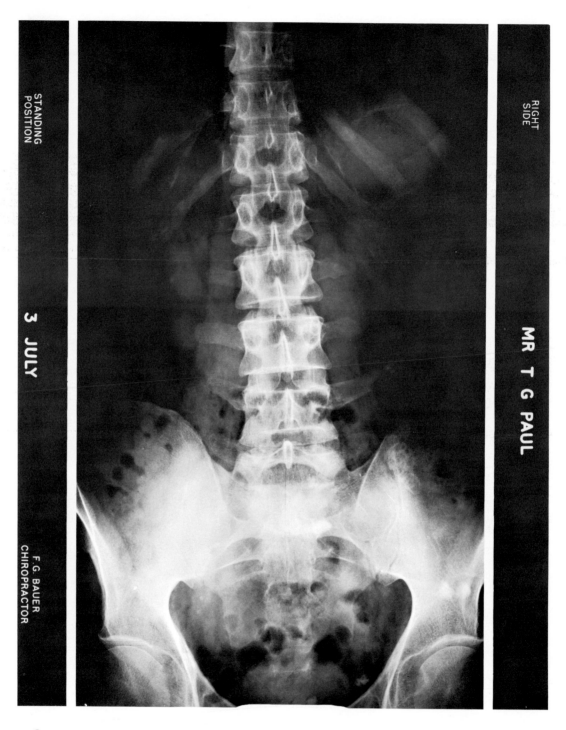

STANDING POSITION

RIGHT SIDE

3 JULY

MR T G PAUL

F.G. BAUER CHIROPRACTOR

C

there is diagnostic value to consider. Any film having black, opaque borders must be easier to read. The absence of strong white light from areas adjacent to information-bearing portions of the film must assist the film reviewer. Still, it is

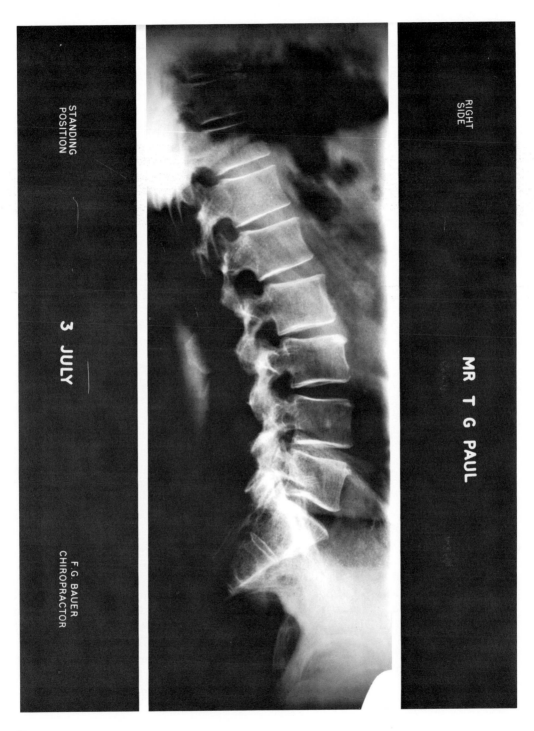

D

understood that this method is time-consuming and only for the aficionado of radiographic excellence. Examples of well-presented films are illustrated in Fig. 10-3.

Exposure Log

There is no doubt that a patient exposure record should be maintained. Basic information is necessary to determine radiation exposure, factor correction, and to maintain accurate records. What follows is a fairly extensive list of items that could appear in an exposure journal; readers may wish to add one or more of these entries to their system of logging exposures.

NAME
AGE
SEX
TELEPHONE NUMBER
DATE
TIME
HEIGHT
WEIGHT
BODY-PART OF INTEREST
VIEW
THICKNESS OF PART
FILM
EXPOSED FILM SIZE
SCREENS
POINTS - refers to points system of
    exposure calculation
FFD
FSD
kVp
mA
mAs
FOCAL SPOT SIZE - if choice exists
FILTERS UTILIZED
GONAD SHIELDS
PREVIOUS AGGREGATE DOSE-
    if information available
SKIN DOSE - nomogram calculated
PERCENTAGE REDUCTION FOR
    FILTERS
BUCKY TIME
DEVELOPMENT TIME
DEVELOPMENT TEMPERATURE
NUMBER OF FILMS - per developer
    lot

TOTAL NUMBER MACHINE
    EXPOSURES
QUALITY - appraisal or estimation
    of film result
RECOMMENDATIONS - if any,
    refers to radiographic quality
REMARKS

Radiographic Copying

There is an increasing demand for "copy films" whether for purposes of referral, study, research or to provide films for mobile patients while maintaining intact records. Copying can be accomplished in the darkroom with the aid of a simple viewbox or with a sophisticated commercial unit. The important point is that an ultraviolet source of light be utilized with copy film.

Copy film has the emulsion on only one side of the film and an anti-halation material on the other side. Halation is the spreading of light, a diffusion process which reduces detail. A veneer of gelatin prevents halation from occurring on the non-emulsion side. The emulsion of copy film is solarized. Originally this meant that a film was exposed to so much sunlight that it altered its "developability." Now film companies solarize film via a chemical process. The practical effect of solarization is that film so treated reacts to light in exactly the opposite manner to that of conventional film. The longer a copy film is exposed to light the lighter it becomes.

Another benefit accruing to copy film users is that of "retouching." An original film may be too dark (dense) in an overall sense. Increasing the exposure time of the copy film will lighten the final film result. With a degree of practice it is even possible to alter portions of a film through "dodging in" and other techniques practiced by adept photographic film processors.

Chapter **11**

Radiation Reduction

No one should ever be allowed to take an x-ray for diagnostic purposes without being able to assess accurately the amount of radiation issued.

F. G. Bauer, 1980

Without fear of contradiction it can be stated that the literature produced concerning the effects of exposure to x-ray would best be measured in tons rather than by any other numerative procedure. The effects of ionizing radiation have been studied almost from the date Roentgen discovered x-ray.

Remarkably, as early as January, 1896, at a clinical congress in Chicago a Dr. Gilman declared that:

". . . any physical agent capable of doing so much damage to normal cells and tissues might offer possibilities if used as a therapeutic agent, in the treatment of a pathological condition in which pronounced irritative blistering or even destructive effects might be desirable."

One E. H. Grubbé, a medical doctor who also manufactured Crookes tubes, suffered from radiation dermatitis as early as January, 1897. Nearly 150 instances of known radiation injury were reported in professional papers by March, 1902. The use and effects of x-ray have been studied

from the beginning and yet unanimity of opinion regarding these effects has not been attained. Does natural radiation exert harmful effects upon genetic tissue? Is there or is there not a linearity of response to radiation? Is there a threshold value beneath which no radiation injury occurs? Just how much radiation-induced chromosomal alteration is repairable? The list of questions could go on for pages. Meanwhile, researchers and authors continue to produce dissonance in the literature while the general public remains largely and blithely unaware of the differences being discussed around it.

One thing is certain. "All ionizing radiation is harmful!" Professor K. Morgan has recently stated that the amount of radiation issued for diagnostic purposes could be reduced to ten percent of its current level without suffering from a loss of information. This direction in thinking is highly desirable, a direction in which we wish all radiation workers were headed. Unfortunately this is not the case. To quote Dr. Morgan on this issue, he declares,

> "I have been endeavoring for over 30 years to point up the need for reducing what I consider is an excessive amount of unnecessary medical exposure to ionizing radiation. The success that I and others have had in these efforts is, to say the least, discouraging when we realize the long way we still have to go . . ."

Radiation should not be handed out like candy at a Christmas party. Please recall to mind the dictum at the beginning of this paragraph when you conduct your next radiologic examination:

> "All ionizing radiation is harmful."

Units of Measurement

Before various aspects of ionizing radiation can be considered the units of radiation measurement must be defined. Discussion will be in terms of the roentgen, the rad and the rem.

In 1974 the International Commission on Radiation Units and Measurements determined that a gradual changeover to SI Units (Systeme Internationale) should take place. With varying degrees of rapidity this process is now occurring.

The roentgen (R) will be replaced by the SI unit of exposure, the coulomb per kilogram (C/kg); the rad will be replaced by the gray (Gy); the international scientific community will replace the rem with the Sievert. Inasmuch as the changeover process will be occurring for several years, and in consideration of the fact that almost all related literature deals in non-SI terms, we have taken what we believe is the logical step of retaining the usage of the earlier units for employment in this book.

The roentgen (R) is the unit of radiation exposure. It occurs in air and so cannot in any way measure the absorbed dose. One roentgen is equal to 2.58×10^{-4} coulomb per kg of air. This definition is quite meaningless to the average x-ray user because it deals in terms which are not related to the clinical application of diagnostic x-ray. While science looks at the roentgen as a precise measurement it is perhaps more useful to consider the roentgen on a comparative basis. In the same way that 60 miles per hour is an absolute speed, it becomes a fast speed when compared to man's walking pace or a slow speed when compared to that of a commercial jetliner. Understanding of the relativities of roentgen and milliroentgen exposures will accompany the progression of written material.

The roentgen is a quantity valuation, not a qualitative assessment. It may be time-related, as in roentgens per hour, but it is not limited to time. Roentgen measurement is free from limitations of field size. Christensen et al explain this feature quite clearly when they equate rainfall and roentgen units. A 1-inch rainfall will yield 1 inch of water in a narrow drinking glass or a broad washtub. So it is with roentgens: the value may apply to an area of 10 square inches or 120 square inches (25 sq. cm or 305 sq. cm).

The rad is an acronym for "radiation absorbed dose." All radiation does not have the same biological effect and the rad helps to correct disparities between tissues. For example, in soft tissue at 50 kVp each rad is 95 percent of the roentgen exposure dose while in bone the rad value is 500 percent of the roentgen figure. This means that a roentgen exposure of 1 R produces an absorbed dose of .95 rad in the skin, a figure of near equivalency. Because the skin dose is so important and because the bone dose is so variable (cortical bone differs from marrow bone; depth and attenuation cause widely varying rad values) the soft tissue ratio of roentgens-to-rads will apply herein. For our purposes then, one roentgen can be considered equal to one rad.

The rem is an acronym for "roentgen equivalent man." This value refers to the biological effect of radiation and takes into consideration a quality factor (QF). The QF of x-rays and gamma rays is one while the QF of protons is five and that of fast neutrons, ten. The equation for determining the rem value is:

Rem = Rads x Quality Factor

The quality factor denotes the effectiveness of specific radiation types in bringing about an equal biological outcome. As in the previous instance when rads are equated with roentgens, because the QF of x-rays is one, rems can be considered equal to rads and roentgens. Therefore, in diagnostic radiation as it relates to the soft tissue/skin dose, it is fair to grade the roentgen, the rad and the rem at parity.

Effects of Radiation

Throughout this book the use of numbered references has been avoided. Now the time for utilizing the investigations, the findings and the thoughts of others is at hand.

Historical Review

In 1896, shortly after the discovery of x-ray a report appeared in the British Medical Journal warning of a dermatitis resulting from radiation [1]. Stanbury [2] suggests that the first attempt to control exposure was put forth by Rollins in 1902 when he advised that radiation which did not fog a photographic plate in seven minutes would not be inimical to man. Sternberg [3] mentions the Boule and Bar account of a severe burn occurring to skin in the abdominal region of a pregnant woman in 1902. This particular woman gave delivery to "apparently healthy twins." Perhaps radiation of low penetrating power was used in this early instance, preventing fetal damage.

The first instance of skin cancer attributed to x-ray was in 1902 and in the following decade almost 100 similar cases were reported in the literature [3]. The use of low energy sources of radiation point to the skin as a highly susceptible tissue. The first time cancer was linked to occupational origin was in 1911 when a case of epidermoid carcinoma on the right hand of a radiologist was reported [4].

Watson [3] points out that radium injections and associated patent medicines were popular in the 1920's and 1930's. In Europe health spas offering radiation came into vogue. The fad was most popular in the United States; a single American clinic apparently administered 14,000 injections of radium. During this period physicians prescribed radium for arthritis, syphilis and mental disorders.

During the late 1920's experiments were conducted with the fruitfly, Drosophilia melanogaster, which revealed that x-ray radiation is capable of producing mutagenesis in tissue cells.

Beginning prior to World War I and continuing through the early 1930's factory workers applied radium-bearing paint to watch faces, producing luminous timepieces. In light of today's knowledge, the workers' habit of placing the tip of the radium-laden brush against their lips to create a precise "point" is absolutely frightening. As could be expected, cases of aplastic anemia, bone sarcomas and carcinomas of the head and paranasal sinuses resulted from this hazardous occupation.

Paralleling the radium dial workers tragedy is that of the therapeutic abortion situation which also occurred from the World War I era until the 1930's. Approximately 350 R were issued to the abdomen of pregnant females and within three to four weeks abortion occurred [5]. Throughout this period radiation-induced abortion was considered to be a harmless and suitable procedure. Occasionally a fetus survived the bombardment, to be born with microcephaly, mental retardation and stunted growth. It is difficult to understand how this nefarious practice was allowed to continue for so many years.

Sternberg located a 1936 report which gave the statistics of a New York City hospital study involving 200 radiation-induced abortions. Miller [6] relates that two reports (1928, 1929) identified a total of 28 cases of disabled infants resulting from pelvic radiotherapy. The ways of science are not always unimpeachable. We shall return later to consideration of the unborn and the child.

Radiologists experienced reduced life spans in the early years of x-ray. Examination of overlapping data in the United States from 1930 until 1958 shows this to be the case, the effects diappearing by 1960 [7]. Early British radiologists did not experience comparable life shortening. However, practice dissimilarities existed between the two countries. Pioneering American radiologists may have accumulated upwards of 2,000 rads [2]. Estimates for exposure to this group of radiologists in 1933 approach 100 R per year while this figure has fallen to 1 R per year by 1957. Japanese x-ray workers are estimated to have been exposed to 900 R per year in 1921, 350 R per year in 1935 and 0.31 R per year after 1958 [4].

Commercial fluoroscopic equipment was widely used in shoe stores for the fitting of footwear up to the 1950's. As radiation protection standards were increased this practice was eliminated. Whether related or not, leukemia mortality rates then dropped for children under 5 years of age. Miller [8] states that 1,000 fewer children died of leukemia between 1960 and 1966 than were expected to when compared with the rate for 1950 to 1959.

A survey of British patients given radiation therapy for ankylosing spondylitis during the 1940's revealed 60 cases of leukemia where 5 cases were expected. Observation of these 14,000 patients continues and final results are not yet known.

Ionizing radiation has been used therapeutically for a dazzling array of benign conditions over the past several decades. A partial list of these conditions follows [9]:

hyperplasia of   hemangiomas
   adenoids   acne

tonsilitis   tinea capitis
mastoiditis   thymic
sinusitis   enlargement
psoriasis   keloids
pruritus ani and lichen simplex
   vulvae   bursitis
peptic ulcer   post-partum
rheumatoid   mastitis
   arthritis   cervical adenitis
eczematous skin
   disease

Radiation was used as a treatment modality for infections until antibiotics came to the forefront in the 1940's. Conditions such as asthma, whooping cough, certain types of deafness and tuberculosis also failed to avoid the therapeutic embrace of ionizing radiation. While no doubt exists in regard to the good intentions of the preceding x-ray users, it can be seen that radiation has been grossly over-utilized in diagnostic and remedial applications. Within the past ten years a well known American radiation authority — who shall remain nameless — stated words to the effect that the sole reason for taking an x-ray is to determine the patient's problem and within broad limits the quantity of radiation issued is irrelevant. It is hoped that all x-ray workers will reject these sentiments as detrimental to the intelligent evolution of safer, saner roentgenology.

Contemporary Review

Of necessity, an overlap of information must occur between historical and contemporary considerations which will, we trust, add to rather than subtract from the continuity of presentation in this section.

The acute lethal effects of x-ray are not of immediate concern to diagnostic radiology. The delayed effects are important and these risks can be categorized as stochastic and non-stochastic effects. Stochastic effects are those which are thought to vary in frequency but not in severity as related to the dose received. There is no known threshold for such effects at current levels of knowledge. Stochastic effects include fetal damage, genetic impairment and carcinogenesis. Non-stochastic effects are dose-related, the severity increasing as the dose increases; a threshold level is considered likely. Non-stochastic effects include decreased fertility, altered hemopoietic activity and cataract formation.

An American survey conducted in 1966 found that 26 percent of 4,071,000 pregnant women had undergone a radiographic examination during the course of their pregnancies. In addition, 11 percent had been exposed to one or more dental x-ray films. Twenty-one percent of these examinations were conducted during the first trimester. Sternberg postulates that the fetus receives between a fraction of 1 rad and 2.5 rads from various radiographic procedures not including, of course, fluoroscopy where exposure levels can be substantially elevated. Morgan[10] discusses the work of Stewart in studying childhood leukemias; fetal doses from diagnostic x-ray were estimated at a surprisingly low 0.3 to 0.8 rad. Early exposure, during the first 18 to 20 days following conception, may lead to expulsion of the ovum. Sufficient irradiation during the the period of organogenesis (days 20 - 50) brings about an impressive array of developmental anomalies which vary according to the stage of fetal growth and level of irradiation. Certainly, at diagnostic levels, the risk increases as the number of films taken increases. It has been suggested that fetal tissue may be 10 times more sensitive to ionizing radiation than adult tissue for comparable exposures.[11]

Various authors and agencies attribute approximately five percent of all childhood malignancies to maternal irradiation at diagnostic x-ray levels. Just as animal tissues may exhibit different response levels to radiation than human tissues, infants and children may vary in susceptibility in comparison to the adult. Children are estimated to be two or three times more liable to contract radiation-induced leukemia than are adults.[6] Survivors of the atomic bomb attacks in Japan provide unfortunate but fruitful opportunities for science to study the effects of ionizing radiation.

The Hiroshima bomb was not the same as the Nagasaki bomb. The active material in the former was uranium which yielded gamma rays and fast neutrons while the latter contained plutonium which produced a preponderance of gamma rays. Data arising from these events are valuable for studying the general effects of ionizing radiation. Leukemia, thyroid carcinoma, lens opacities and growth irregularities are conditions generally agreed to have increased in frequency due to post-natal or intra-uterine exposure resulting from atomic bombings of the Japanese. The Hiroshima and Nagasaki episodes were planned situations; the Marshall Islands affair was an accident.

In 1954 a thermonuclear device was exploded on Bikini Island, regrettably causing heavy fallout exposure to the native population, particularly residents of Rongelap Island. Of the 19 children less than 10 years old at the time of the accident, all have since developed thyroid abnormalities. From a dose estimated at a maximum of 175 R, growth retardation, increased incidence of miscarriage and lymphocytic chromosomal irregularities have occurred.[7]

Key words consistently appear in the literature: "thyroid carcinoma," "children" and "leukemia" are in every vocabulary of radiation damage. Even in consideration of benign nodules of the thyroid, it seems that children are two or three times more susceptible than are adults to induction of these nodules by radiation.[12] Foster [13] reported that children with thyroid carcinoma had a history of prior irradiation in up to 75 or 80 percent of cases studied. He also postulated that a child receiving 200 R to the thyroid would have a one percent chance of developing thyroid carcinoma within 20 years. (Certain scanning procedures could result in the thyroid receiving 65 to 90 R in a single diagnostic examination.) In discussing risk estimates Brown [14] reviewed the findings of Gibson et al (1972) wherein the chance of developing acute or chronic myeloid leukemia is two to three times higher in men who "received 21 or more diagnostic films to the trunk . . . and as much as seven-fold higher in men who received 41 or more films."

Fry and Ainsworth [15] examined the factors which influence risk estimates in carcinogenesis. The physical factors influencing tumor induction are:

Dose
Dose Rate
Fractionation
Protraction
Radiation Quality

We believe it is important to realize that there has been a significant quantitive modification in many of these factors over the years. Doses that were thought to be safe in 1940 were disowned in 1960 and positively shunned by 1980. Dose rates that were permissible in sundry jurisdictions are now looked at askance by radiation workers. There are no compelling reasons to assume that radiation protection standards have reached their apogee.

What sort of doses put an individual at risk? The National Academy of Science — National Research Council, Subcommittee on Somatic Effects, calculated that an additional 0.1 rem (whole-body) exposure to the U.S. population could cause 1,350 to 3,300 additional deaths annually. Morgan [10] refers to the Bross findings: various population groups experience increased susceptibility to radiation damage. For example, children already suffering from asthma, hives, eczema, allergy, pneumonia, rheumatic fever and other diseases have shown leukemia susceptibility up to 50 times above expectations following x-ray exposure.

Between 1949 and 1960 a total of 11,000 Israeli youths were irradiated for tinea capitis. Studies indicate that as little as six to nine rads can be tumorogenic to the thyroid gland. [8, 10, 14, 16] Surprisingly, while x-ray irradiation was utilized as a tinea treatment modality for 50 years no research was conducted pertaining to the late effects of this therapy. The first such report was issued in 1968 when thyroid malignancies were discovered in a group of treated children. Harley et al [17] carried out further tests via thermoluminescent dosimetry and found that the average thyroid dose from typical epilation treatment totaled 6±2 rads. The same therapy has been observed to induce salivary gland carcinoma and brain tumors, particularly meningioma. Upton [18] notes that the "estimated risks per unit dose" were not less in children receiving 6 or 7 rads than in those receiving 100 or 200 and more rads. Because of widely varying sensitivity of tissues to the induction of malignancy through radiation many of the old "safe" doses are now hazardous. Upton contends that other cancers, of protracted latency periods, may as yet be unknown to those investigating induction of neoplasia via irradiation. Radiation-induced thyroid carcinoma has been observed to have a latency period of 4 to 29 years. It can readily be seen that exposures of the head and neck must be undertaken with all due care and consideration.

Brown [14] believes that in considering breast cancer, leukemia and thyroid carcinoma there is not a lower risk per rad at lower doses. Instead, he asserts that published data favor a higher risk per rad at low doses as compared to high doses.

In the preceding "Historical Review" we looked at irradiation for benign conditions. What does today's literature tell us about these activities? A study was done of 5,000-plus children who were irradiated between 1935 and 1955 for certain benign conditions especially in the cervicocranial region. Upon recall examination in the 1970's these individuals revealed a 24 percent incidence of palpable thyroid nodules or altered thyroid activity.[19] Apparently investigators are developing a recall program to canvas youths who underwent fluoroscopic examinations in Seattle, Washington, during the 1940's and 1950's. During these years a group of five pediatricians examined children via fluoroscopy and allowed the mothers to watch. Sometimes infants were even examined each month for the first year. Whole-body radiation received has been estimated to range from 5 R per minute to 60 R per minute. A paper by Degroot and Paloyan is discussed in Sloan's article [16] wherein thyroid carcinoma is referred to as a "Chicago endemic." It was found that 40 percent of thyroid cancer cases at the University of Chicago Hospital from 1968-1972 had undergone radiation therapy, most often for benign disorders. A further 100 asymptomatic individuals who had experienced similar irradiation were examined. Twenty-six percent had thyroid tumors of which seven proved to be malignant. In another Chicago hospital recall program of prodigious proportions, 1,500 examinations were conducted; thyroid tumors were found in 27 percent of those investigated. Surgical intervention resulted in a diagnosis of carcinoma for one-third of this study group, or an apparent nine percent incidence of thyroid carcinoma in irradiated subjects.

Leukemia is the most common x-ray-induced neoplasm encountered in man. However, it is not always easy to link irradiation to tumor induction because such neoplasms are "clinically indistinguishable from those which occur spontaneously."[20] Stanbury [2] converts International Commission on Radiological Protection figures to everyday values: ". . . there is one chance in 50,000 of inducing leukemia in a patient who receives 1 rad of bone marrow radiation." Over a period of 20 to 25 years post-

exposure, Bond expects the leukemia risk to entail 20 additional cases per million exposed people per rad of exposure.[21]

Children receiving radiation for thymic enlargement undergo a thyroid cancer risk estimated at 2.5 excess cases for each million children exposed to 1 rad per year.[22] The BEIR Report (Report of the Advisory Committee on Biological Effects of Ionizing Radiation, National Academy of Sciences — National Research Council) extrapolated high dose irradiation data to low dose estimates. They suggest that diagnostic levels of radiation to the United States population in the amount of 0.1 R per person per year would result in 2,000 to 9,000 cancer deaths per year.

Non-stochastic effects receive less attention in the literature, as could be expected. For example, most x-ray workers accept a value of 200 to 500 rads as being the minimal threshold for induction of lens opacities. Similar situations exist for alterations in the hemopoietic picture. Modifications in fertility have been documented through studies of animals. It remains for us to briefly review genetic changes, the one stochastic effect not yet addressed.

Genetic mutations are of two types:
1. Point mutations
2. Chromosomal aberrations

Biochemical alterations within DNA material occur in point mutations. The result is an alteration in the genetic code. The effect varies from minor to lethal and the majority of recessive mutations are thought to occur in point mutations. Chromosomal aberrations display damage, breakage or rearrangement of chromosomal material. There does not appear to be a threshold level beneath which radiation-induced mutations fail to occur.

An exposure as low as 12 rads following diagnostic roentgenology has resulted in chromosomal alterations in man. Further, similar changes have been seen in radiation workers receiving an average of 1.4 rems per year. A dose of 1.5 to 2 R per year over a 30-year period will create generous numbers of mutations to the gene pool of a country's population.[23] It has been stated that 0.1 percent or less of all mutations are beneficial. Bearing this figure in mind, the potential for retrograde genetic alterations through ionizing radiation may be comprehended. There is no doubt that radiation increases the production of mutations both in animals and man.

In concluding this abbreviated exercise reviewing the effects of radiation, a quote from Dr. K. Z. Morgan [24] is appropriate:

> "During the past 25 years, however, there has accumulated a preponderance of evidence which indicates there is no safe threshold dose and in fact both experimental and theoretical evidence seem to indicate there is no dose or dose rate of ionizing radiation so low that the risk of radiation damage is zero."

Environmental Radiation

Radiation has been with humanity from time immemorial, possibly causing effects even to earliest man. It is well for us to consider this source of x-ray radiation for its consequences are so diverse as to range from affecting a box of radiographic film in the darkroom of an x-ray user to the possibility of altering the history of mankind. Presently, aspects of environmental radiation will be considered and this will be followed in the next section by procedures to estimate radiation exposure levels from diagnostic roentgenology.

Society is concerned about oil spillages at sea and the possible detrimental effects of these episodes. What must also be taken into consideration is the continual seepage of oil from the sea bed into the oceans of the world. A similar situation arises in regard to radiation. Measures to limit ionizing radiation from man-made sources are certainly important. However, the effect background radiation plays upon genetic and somatic consequences

provides tantalizing food for thought. The National Academy of Sciences — National Research Council (U.S.) postulates that one percent of spontaneous carcinomas in America are caused by background radiation, a figure amounting to 3,000 to 4,000 deaths each year. Their "guesstimate" may prove to be quite inaccurate in the years ahead. Nevertheless, it is a starting point and does illustrate the need for further research, including epidemiological studies.

Americans receive an estimated 180 millirems of radiation exposure per year, roughly 100 millirems originating from environmental sources and 80 millirems from medical and diagnostic x-ray sources.[25] The latter portion of this aggregate radiation varies markedly from country to country, citizens of less developed nations of course receiving much less exposure.

Natural background radiation alters from area to area and even the altitude of the region influences exposure levels. Dunedin, New Zealand receives 37 millirems per year from natural sources while Rome, Italy receives 180 millirems.[3] Inhabitants of Denver, Colorado receive approximately twice as much cosmic radiation at their residential height of one mile as do inhabitants of sea-level cities. Residents of La Paz, Bolivia receive approximately four times the cosmic radiation usually experienced at sea-level sites. The curious reader may wonder what happens to radiation levels during an airplane flight. The answer is that levels rise sharply: at 32,000 feet cosmic radiation is twelve times that of the value at sea-level.[26] Ostensibly, the duration of commercial flights is such that no danger is posed, even for the pregnant woman.

Two areas of the world have unusually high levels of radiation which arise from ground sources. A portion of Brazil has black sands comprising in part, monazite and ilmenite which produce radiation levels up to 5mR/hr on the surface of the sands. Monazite contains 5 to 10 percent of a radioactive element, thorium. (Regional tourists vacation in the area to obtain the therapeutic benefits of the well-known black sands!) The nearby city of Guarapari experiences ten times the normal levels of background radiation.[27] Monazite deposits are distributed more widely in Kerala, India, where 100,000 natives are exposed to radiation varying from 0.2 to 2.6 R/yr. To date no large-scale epidemiological studies have been conducted on residents of these areas. Therefore, little knowledge exists pertaining to the effects of these naturally occurring elevated levels of radioactivity.

Buildings themselves give off radioactivity which presents implications for the x-ray user beyond the effects of these emissions upon man. Increased levels of radiation may readily fog unexposed radiographic film which has not been kept adequately protected within lead-lined storage containers. A fascinating article concerning this subject was written by a Swedish x-ray worker, Arne Lundh.[28] The background radiation from many building materials is considerably elevated in Sweden and this peculiarity proves troublesome to numerous x-ray installations. The radioactive potassium, thorium and radium content in many local mineral building materials causes varying degrees of film fogging. For example, wood is nearly free of radioactivity whereas certain types of Swedish concrete blocks or granite may emit 1.2 mR/day. The type of ray that causes "building material fogging" is the gamma ray; the resultant fog alters the potential film density, the average contrast of the film and the film speed. Lundh believes proper shielding for films is far more significant in controlling fog than is cold storage, a well regarded fog-restraining measure.

The human body even contributes to its own radiation dose, depending on individual diet and metabolism. Natural potassium within the body contains a minute fraction of radioactive potassium which delivers a dose to the gonads in the order of 20 to 25 millirems per year. It has been suggested that the body contributes to its own carcinogenesis via self-irradiation, although no evidence supporting this contention has been discovered. [26]

There are few certainties in the x-ray world when it comes to either late genetic or late somatic effects of irradiation. It is known, however, that radiation is not beneficial to constituent tissues of the human body. The environmental/natural portion of our annual dosage cannot really be avoided: moving from Rome to Dunedin does not seem to be a pragmatic solution to an indeterminate problem. Thus, if we are to keep the aggregate exposure of ourselves and our fellow men to what is currently accepted as a safe level of irradiation, we must do all within our power to lessen the man-made contribution of ionizing radiation, not just for today but for every day.

Calculating Radiation

Webster's definition of "calculate" includes a differentiation between 'calculate,' 'compute,' 'estimate' and 'reckon.' "Calculate" is the preferred term when dealing with a "highly intricate process" where the answer is open to question "rather than exact or definite" in kind. Calculation of radiation certainly is intricate and its assessment borders on the problematical. Calculation of radiation is an important yet oft-neglected area of knowledge for many health professionals and/or x-ray users. It is important that an individual health professional who is requesting x-ray services realizes what his/her patient is receiving in the way of radiation dosage before the study is ordered. It is important for the x-ray worker to be aware of radiation dosages so that the safest techniques, equipment and technology can be implemented. The health professional who is also an x-ray user has a moral obligation to prescribe no more views than are clinically necessary and then to insure that all due care is exercised in every facet of radiographic practice. Learning how to calculate radiation is necessary to a fuller understanding of its use. That having been said, we now are able to proceed to the actual calculation of radiation, albeit not in a straight-line advance.

There are too many variables to allow for the precise determination of radiation dosages. In the first place, we must speak of estimating radiation exposures, not radiation dosages. Earlier in this chapter roentgens, rads and rems were graded at parity insofar as skin doses are concerned. For practical purposes in diagnostic radiology this is quite true. Nevertheless, the reader must realize that the *nomogram* measures radiation in terms of exposure, which is the roentgen unit.

By definition, a nomogram uses a straightedge to measure a variable which has been plotted through knowledge of two (or more) independent variables. The nomogram provides the simplest, most easily utilized method of calculating radiation for everyday purposes. No x-ray facility should be without one. The surface exposure nomogram needs only two input factors — kVp and FSD — to produce a reasonably accurate exposure dose in roentgen values.

The calculation of radiation is not totally precise because no two x-ray machines are exactly alike. There are several reasons for deviation from the standard:

(1) Voltage wave form variations occur in the high tension transformer. Also included in this category are differences in losses from the copper and iron cores.
(2) Filament transformers experience variations in efficiency.
(3) Supply line disparities occur in different machines and in the same machine at different times.
(4) The efficiency of an x-ray tube

varies as to its age, use, amount of focal track roughening, etc.

We have consulted several previously prepared nomograms and compared the values obtained for like exposures. As can be gathered from the reasons stated above, the readings varied appreciably. In an attempt to update and improve upon earlier efforts we determined to produce a new nomogram. For convenience in preparation, it was decided to base the nomogram upon the F. G. Bauer x-ray installation. The radiation branch of the Health Commission of New South Wales co-operated fully, sending technical personnel on several occasions to perform exposure readings and to assist with and to verify test methods. The results of these tests are summarized in Appendix A.

Using the Nomogram

Please refer to the surface exposure nomogram reproduced in Fig. 11-1. The top line refers to the focus-skin distance. The bottom line represents the kVp employed. Two mm of aluminum filtration is the amount of added filtration commonly used in modern equipment. The area labeled "no filter" at the lower aspect of the bottom line reveals just how much more radiation reaches the subject when filtration is omitted. The middle line assigns a milliroentgens per milliampere seconds value to the exposure in question. For example, suppose that a particular exposure produced 5 mR/mAs and that the exposure amounted to 100 mAs. Thus, the exposure is 100 x 5 = 500 mR or 0.5 R.

As long as values can be obtained for the top and bottom scales, the middle scale can be calculated by locating the mR/mAs value and multiplying by the mAs for a particular film exposure. The easiest way of locating the middle line reference point is with a piece of fine black thread or string. Drawn tautly between the kVp and FSD lines, the milliroentgens per milliampere second

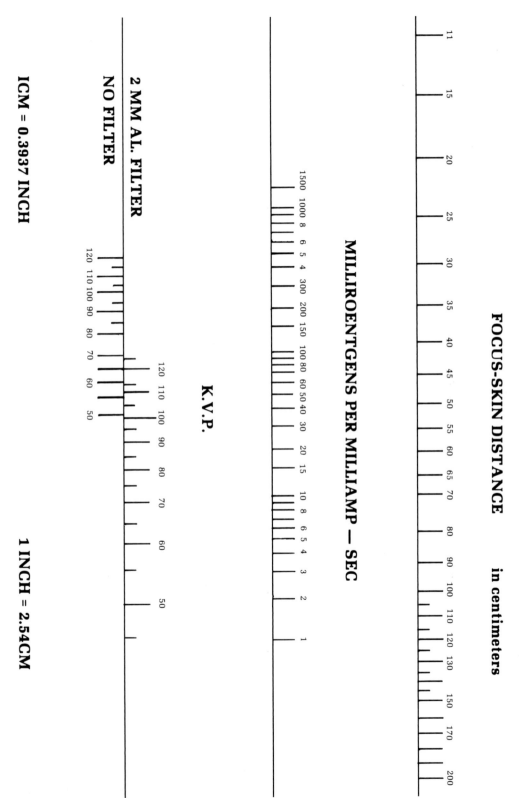

Fig. 11-1 — Surface exposure nomogram

value is easily read. Another suitable measure to locate co-ordinates accurately is a clear plastic or acrylic rule with a fine black line drawn on it.

Example No. 1

An A-P lumbar imaging examination is conducted at 100 kVp, 50 mAs, 100cm FFD and the patient is 22cm thick. Allowing 3cm for the bucky apparatus (The subject is 3cm away from the film because of the intevening bucky and therefore 3cm closer to the tube.) The FSD is 75cm. The nomogram reveals that the line between 100 kVp and 75cm FSD yields approximately 15 mR/mAs. The tube exposure is 50 mAs, producing a total of 750 mR or 0.75 R.

$$15 \text{ mR/mAs} \times 50 \text{ mAs} = 750 \text{ mR}$$

This has been a purely hypothetical exercise bearing no relevance beyond that of becoming comfortable with using the nomogram. We shall move ahead to comparative examples, illustrating how radiation dosages differ according to the exposure techniques used.

Example No. 2

A lateral lumbosacral examination of a patient 33cm in thickness is conducted, employing the following factors:

Recommended Exposure Technique:
   kVp - 100
   mAs - 400
   FFD - 200cm
   FSD - 165cm (2cm allowed for patient-to-film distance)

Result:
   $3 \text{ mR/mAs} \times 400 \text{ mAs} = 1,200 \text{ mR}$ or 1.2 R

Example No. 3

A lateral lumbosacral examination of a patient 33cm in thickness is conducted using a conventional exposure technique. The FFD is usually shortened to 100cm and the kVp is significantly lessened.

Conventional Exposure Technique:
   kVp - 85

mAs - 300
FFD - 100cm
FSD - 163cm (4cm allowed for patient-to-film distance)

Result:
   $17 \text{ mR/mAs} \times 300 \text{ mAs} = 5,100 \text{ mR}$ or 5.1 R

The high/optimal kilovoltage technique in conjunction with a 200cm FFD clearly issues much less radiation to the patient. By way of explanation, it should be noted that the exposure techniques for Examples Nos. 2 and 3 did not come from a hypothetical technique chart. The factors came from actual machine installations, Example No. 3 resulting from a survey conducted among several local hospitals and radiologic installations. Also, it should be noted that 4cm was allowed for the (table-top) patient-to-film distance in the conventional technique because buckys used in recumbent table work often allow a gap of 4cm or more between the patient and the film. In fact, gaps of 10cm are not unusual.

The radiation calculations in the previous three examples have been determined "free-in-air" at the skin surface. This is expressed as Exposure at Skin Entrance (ESE) and is stated in milliroentgens. Example No. 1 is correctly read as an ESE of 750 mR. To proceed a step further and obtain a more realistic assessment of the amount of radiation issued, a backscatter factor must be added to the computed estimate. The skin surface receives not only direct radiation from the x-ray tube; it also receives a contribution of scattered radiation. Appendix B lists the backscatter factors for several common films which have been collimated to useful field sizes.

Returning to Example No. 1 once again, an A-P lumbar film can be collimated to 10″ x 17″. In most instances collimation will improve the diagnostic value of the film in normal circumstances. The backscatter factor for a 10″ x 17″ film at 100 kVp is 1.40. Taking the original figure of

750 mR and multiplying it by 1.40 gives a total surface exposure of 1,050 mR or 1.05 R.

750 mR x 1.40 Backscatter Factor = 1,050 mR

Example No. 4
An A-P cervical examination of a patient 13cm in thickness is conducted with the following factors.

    kVp - 100
    mAs - 125
    FFD - 200cm
    FSD - 185cm
          (2cm allowed for bucky)
Result:

    2.3 mR/mAs x 125 mAs =
            287.5 mR(ESE)

In this example high-definition screens are used. If faster calcium tungstate or rare-earth screens are employed the exposure dose would be even less.

The backscatter factor for a film collimated to 5″ x 10″ is 1.35 at 100 kVp. Thus, the total exposure at the skin surface is 388 mR.

Skin Surface:
The final subject matter to be considered in regard to calculating radiation is the body's skin surface. There are complex formulae which can be used to compute the skin surface of an individual. Obviously, the skin surface area of an obese male 6′ (183cm) in height will differ from that of a slender male 5′6″ (168cm) in height. The volume of tissue is, of course, a consideration and while the larger individual has a greater skin surface he also has a greater volume of tissue subject to irradiation. Nevertheless, attempting to train health professionals to the level of computer programmers will only discourage the adoption of radiation calculation procedures. Moreover, an average figure will suffice for normal comparative purposes.

The average male skin surface is 18,000 sq. cm
The average female skin surface is 16,000 sq. cm
The average infant skin surface is 2,200 sq. cm

The international recommendation for overall allowable skin exposure is not to exceed 0.5 R per year for non-radiation workers, i.e., patients. On this basis collimated field sizes can be related to the entire body surface. If the field size of a particular view is ten percent of the entire body surface and that view yields 5,000 mR (5 R), then no further radiographs can be taken for a year without exceeding the international recommendation for man-made radiation.

Example No. 5
A 14″ x 17″ (35cm x 43cm) A-P lumbar film of a female is collimated to the actual film size. In round figures this collimated area represents ten percent of the total skin surface. If the total skin surface is allowed 0.5 R then one-tenth, or ten percent, of the skin surface is allowed 5 R. Suppose that the exposure yielded 2.0 R for this area; this means that only one more like radiograph could be taken in one year. Two more like exposures would exceed international recommendations.

The chart reproduced in Fig. 11-2 is a compilation of several common film sizes and collimated areas, providing skin surface percentages and annual "allowable" radiation exposures. Male and female skin surfaces have been averaged for ease of application. Collimated areas have been converted from inches to centimeters to facilitate calculations involving body skin surfaces, which are quoted in centimeters. Each collimated film size comprises a percentage of the total skin surface; e.g., one 10″ x 17″ exposure of the average male embraces 6.1 percent of his total skin surface.

The last column provides the amount (in roentgens) to which a specific area can be exposed without exceeding the internationally recommended value of 0.5 R annually for the entire skin surface. For example, in the male an 8″ x 10″ area

FIG. 11-2

RELATIONSHIP OF SKIN SURFACE TO RADIATION

MALE-18,000 SQ. CM.

Collimated Film Size	Percentage of Skin Surface	Max. Annual Allowable Exposure per Area
1. 5" x 10" = 323cm²	1.8	27.9 R
2. 8" x 10" = 516cm²	2.9	17.4 R
3. 6" x 17" = 658cm²	3.7	13.7 R
4. 7" x 17" = 768cm²	4.3	11.7 R
5. 10" x 17" = 1097cm²	6.1	8.2 R
6. 14" x 17" = 1536cm²	8.5	5.9 R
7. 14" x 36" = 3252cm²	18.1	2.8 R

FEMALE-16,000 SQ. CM.

Collimated Film Size	Percentage of Skin Surface	Max. Annual Allowable Exposure per Area
1. 5" x 10" = 323cm²	2.0	24.8 R
2. 8" x 10" = 516cm²	3.2	15.5 R
3. 6" x 17" = 658cm²	4.1	12.2 R
4. 7" x 17" = 768cm²	4.8	10.4 R
5. 10" x 17" = 1097cm²	6.9	7.3 R
6. 14" x 17" = 1536cm²	9.6	5.2 R
7. 14" x 36" = 3252cm²	20.3	2.5 R

can receive 17.4 R before exceeding international recommendations, providing no other areas are examined. Thus, if one 8" x 10" view yields 0.5 R, a total of 35 like films could be taken before the annual whole-body radiation recommendation is exceeded, again providing of course that no other films are taken in other areas. If a 14" x 36" film is being considered, the area must not receive more than 2.5 R in the female or 2.8 R in the male. If respective single views receive 2.5 R or 2.8 R then no other films may be taken during the next year without exceeding agreed limits.

Note the percentage of skin surface exposed by the 14" x 36" view. In the female this amounts to 20.5 percent of the total and in the male it is 18.1 percent. Compare this figure with the percentage of skin surface exposed by 7" x 17" and 10" x 17" films and one can see why stringent collimation is such an important part of any radiation control program.

The examples given above also illustrate why it is most important to keep retake rates at a minimum. A responsible approach to radiology necessitates the x-ray user being conversant with radiation calculation procedures and utilizing this information in workaday conditions. The definitive question concerning radiation calculation is as follows:

> If an x-ray user cannot calculate radiation exposures, how then can that individual assess various radiographic techniques and how then will that individual be able to adopt measures which yield *less* radiation?

Comparison of X-Ray Machines:

> To compare the radiation output of another single-phase fully rectified x-ray machine with that of the unit used as the basis for the nomogram printed herein, at least two readings should be made by qualified personnel with properly calibrated radiation measuring equipment. Any deviation (+ or -) from the calculated results appearing in the nomogram should be figured in percentages, thereafter each calculation being corrected by the same percentage factor.

Reducing Radiation

It is manifestly obvious that x-ray is detrimental to living tissue. Exposures so small as to produce no demonstrable biological effect have yet to be produced. Like automobiles, airplanes, and a host of other creations of modern civilization, diagnostic x-rays possess capabilities for great good and for great harm to societies and to individuals. In order to maintain the balance scales so that benefits outweigh risks, radiation levels to mankind must be reduced. Fortunately, this task can be advanced by x-ray users everywhere, beginning today. Sometimes great expenditures of funds are necessary to meet objectives. In other instances no monetary resources are needed to reach desired goals; increased knowledge, greater care and amplified motivation often work wonders. There are quite literally dozens of things that can be done to improve radiographic quality and lessen radiation dosages at the same time. A partial list of these items and activities is presented. Any x-ray user

conscientiously applying the ten factors enumerated will be performing a major service to his/her patients.

1. Accurate Collimation

Forget the fact that governments are instituting mandatory automatic beam collimation. There are innumerable instances where collimation can be restricted beyond that which is required by law. Scatter radiation diminishes as the area irradiated contracts. The volume of tissue irradiated also diminishes with tightened collimation because the size of the area under examination determines the volume of tissue exposed. As scatter depends upon tissue volume, contrast likewise is improved by small field sizes. Always collimate stringently.

2. Optimal kVp

Spinal studies performed at 82 kVp or 75 kVp or even lower are no longer acceptable from a radiation standpoint. Yes, increased scatter is produced at higher kVp levels. However, a corresponding reduction in radiation dosages at higher kilovoltages mandates the adoption of optimal kilovoltage techniques. Increasing kilovoltage increases the penetrating power of the x-ray beam. We are firmly convinced that diagnostic spinal procedures are best undertaken at 100 kVp in almost all instances. It is not true that scatter causes problems at 100 kVp if other exposure considerations are maintained at correct levels. It is true that 100 kVp makes a substantial improvement in radiation reduction when compared to the factors utilized in a 75 kVp technique. Yes, contrast is less at 100 kVp than at lower kilovoltages but it is never decreased to an unsatisfactory dimension by kVp alone. Other factors must be at fault for this to occur.

3. Minimal mAs

Milliamperage controls the number of x-ray photons produced during an exposure. If the mAs is high, many photons reach the patient. Stated simply, increased milliamperage gives rise to an increased patient dosage. A high kilovoltage technique requires less milliamperage to obtain the same film density; hence high kilovoltage is the method of choice for reduced radiation levels.

4. Maximum Focus Film Distance

It is surprising how often one comes across individuals who still believe that short FFD's mean shorter exposure times (true) and therefore lowered radiation dosages (false). A short FFD leads to greater radiation levels reaching the patient, all through the mandates of the Inverse Square Law, as discussed in Chapter I. An ideal distance for spinal studies is 200cm (80") — penumbra is reduced, magnification and distortion are diminished and radiation levels are curtailed. A brief return to the nomogram will illustrate the degree of ensuing radiation reduction.

5. Proficient Grid

The question may well be asked: "How does a grid play a role in radiation reduction? That's like saying a small focal spot or automatic processing lessens radiation. It is patently untrue." In the strict sense the inclusion of grids amongst radiation reduction factors does deserve scrutiny. The use of a grid improves film contrast but only at the expense of increased patient exposure. However, unless a satisfactory grid is used film clarity suffers from excess secondary scatter radiation, lessening the diagnostic value of the film(s). Of even more importance is the inability to use high kilovoltage or long FFD techniques without the supportive benefits of a quality bucky-grid combination. Not infrequently x-ray users will attempt to use an 8:1 grid in conjunction with 100 kVp, only to be disappointed by poor results. Grids must be adequate for the task at hand which, in our recommendations, means employing a 12:1 grid for 100 kVp use, or a 16:1 model for applications at higher kilovoltages. It is worth mentioning again that grids with aluminum interspacing offer additional clean-up properties without requiring an augmentation of either kVp or mAs.

6. Fastest Appropriate Screens

By using any screen at all the patient experiences a reduced radiation exposure. Using the fastest screen possible, commensurate with the requirements of the examination being performed, lessens radiation to the lowest practical level. Of course this does not mean using the fastest rare-earth screen in combination with a fast film so that quantum mottle destroys the diagnostic value of a film. It does mean keeping up with developments in screen technology, a rapidly evolving area of radiography, so that exposure reductions can be made as refinements permit. Quite often screen speed rises faster than resolving power falls. That is, screen speed may go up 100 per cent while loss of resolution may fall 60 to 70 percent, an overall gain. As long as quality imaging standards are maintained the faster screens are acceptable.

7. Correct Filtration

Filtration is considered in two equally important classifications:

1. Correct added filtration
2. Correct density equalizing filtration (DEF)

For our purposes added filtration includes the inherent filtration of the tube and its appurtenances. This means that there must be sufficient filtration for the beam to be effectively "hardened" for all exposures. It would be criminal — and highly illegal — to use a 100kVp technique in conjunction with a total of 1mm aluminum filtration. Whether thicknesses of aluminum or half-value layers (HVL) are the standard of measurement, added filtration is necessary to remove low-energy radiation which does nothing positive for the final film result but which certainly does harm the patient.

Density equalizing filtration is a boon to patients undergoing diagnostic spinal examinations. In lateral lumbar studies there is no reason in the wide world that T12-L1 should receive the same amount of radiation that L5-S1 receives; L5 area is difficult to penetrate, L1 area is usually easy to penetrate. Further, there is no reason why a lateral lumbar "spot" view is necessary if DEF is employed. An A-P cervicothoracic view on 17" (43cm) film is appropriate with DEF; without it the same view quite often is a disaster. In general, properly designed and applied filtration is of very real benefit in both diagnostic and dosage considerations.

8. Correct Processing

Processing is far more important to radiation dosages than one might think, with either manual or automatic processing regimes. Deep-tank developing with understrength, weakened or improperly replenished solutions is a sure cause of patient overexposure. Automatic processing with diluted developer or inadequate temperature control is likewise a harbinger of excess patient irradiation. The time-worn aphorism which states that "Radiography begins and ends in the darkroom" is a well founded guide for all x-ray users.

9. Suitable Film

As the remnant beam exits the patient being examined, the information which will later appear on film is at the stage of maximum availability. If this information is imprinted upon slow, finegrain film then maximum retrieval of information occurs; however, increased radiation levels also occur. The slow film requires more photons to energize the film's emulsion constituents. A fast coarse-grained film retrieves much less information than slow varieties but radiation levels are minimized.

The film used should be as fast as possible while still meeting the requirements necessary to produce a thoroughly diagnostic result. Films and screens can detract from diagnostic results if the components are incorrect, or are incorrectly matched. Usually the most satisfactory film-screen combination is a medium or par speed film used in conjunction with a fast screen. Technology promises further developments in the application of films and screens and so the preceding recommendation may alter in the foreseeable future.

10. Bilateral Compression & Gonadal Shields

The bilateral compression band immobilizes the patient, which is a diagnostically sound practice in conventional spinal studies. It decreases the thickness of the patient in A-P lumbosacralpelvic views, allowing for a reduced radiation dosage through lessened factors.

Properly applied, the gonadal shields—which attach to the BCB—reduce radiation dosages to the related male and female germinative tissue by more than 90 percent. Surely there can be no other single item which is so easily applied, so remarkably inexpensive and which does so much to lessen radiation exposure to a critical area. Gonadal shielding deserves to come into general usage almost immediately and to be decreed mandatory within a reasonable period of time. Unfortunately, as with the wearing of seat belts, few jurisdictions are willing to enact regulations that save lives if those rules impinge upon individual or professional conduct.

Radiation can be reduced by taking fewer views of an area, which is especially important when critical structures are included within the field of view. The maximum number of films of an area often is not the optimal number of films necessary for diagnosis. Transferring films between professional users of diagnostic radiology whenever studies and views compatible for the needs at hand makes eminently good sense. Repeat examinations for administrative rather than clinical reasons are to be eschewed as inimical to the best interest of the patient. Periodic inspections of radiographic equipment by the user and by outside service personnel helps to maintain a high standard of operating efficiency. Up-to-date equipment (of ample capacity) is the only type suitable for any x-ray user.

All of the above measures reduce patient exposure to ionizing radiation. These, and other measures, should be studied, evaluated and put into effect where there are areas of weakness in an x-ray facility.

Practical Perspective

"HOW MUCH RADIATION EXPOSURE
DID THIS PATIENT ACTUALLY RECEIVE?"

How much radiation exposure did this patient actually receive? The lateral lumbar spine film illustrated also includes the entire sacrum and coccyx and the lowest four thoracic vertebrae. The sketch of this area reveals the coverage of the filtration employed during the exposure.

Density equalizing filtration is superimposed over areas (A), (B) and (C). An ovarian shield protects area (E) while area (D) receives the emergent beam unfiltered beyond the anterior surface of the collimator. (A) and (B) are screened respectively by filters 4 and 5, the diaphragm and back-scatter filters. Filtration in both instances is laminated: 1.5mm aluminum on either side of a core of 1mm copper. Area (C) is shielded by one of the wedge filters, in this instance filter 1, i.e., 3mm aluminum. Filter 1 also overlies all of (A) and almost all of (B).

As stated, area (D) is not the recipient of any Density Equalizing Fltration whereas (E) is protected by a lead gonadal shield of 3mm lead thickness.

The skin exposure, measured "free-in-air", was obtained with an electrometer manufactured by Electronic Instruments Ltd., Richmond, England, and was taken by a representative of the radiation branch of the Health Commission of New

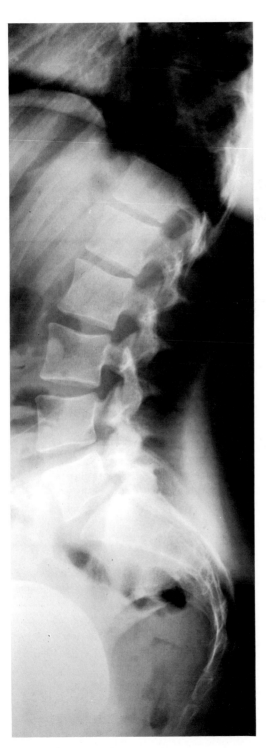

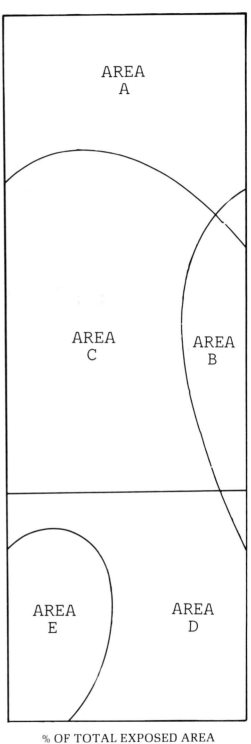

Practical Perspective

% OF TOTAL EXPOSED AREA

A + B	=	36%
C	=	36%
D	=	22%
E	=	6%
TOTAL % 100		

South Wales. The exposure over area (D) was 0.37 R. (Remarks made in Chapter XI concerning exact, absolute measurements of radiation apply equally here.) Using a surface nomogram figures were calculated for the remaining areas. These areas (A) and (B) received 0.02 R, or 5.64 percent of (D); (C) received 0.188 R, 50.81 percent of (D); (E) received 0.000 R, or zero percent of (D). Filtration resulted in a radiation exposure reduction of 58.6 percent in this instance. It can be stated that in general an average reduction of 50 percent occurs through the use of DEF in the lateral lumbar spine examination.

Particulars of the exposure concerned in this depiction are as follows. The patient was a 30-year-old female, 30cm thickness, exposed at 100 kVp and 160 mAs over a focus-film distance of 200cm. Dupont Hi-Plus screens were employed in conjunction with 2 DC radiographic film, the final result obtained through manual deep-tank processing.

There is no doubt that Density Equalizing Filtration is efficacious in reducing radiation. The conscientious x-ray user should regard filtration as an integral component of the radiodiagnostic armamentarium.

While we have repeatedly stressed radiation reduction, our attention to this topic has been positive rather than negative. All x-ray users can reduce radiation dosages issued to patients; all x-ray users can assist in mitigating the potentially harmful effects of radiation; all x-ray users can provide an improved service to their patients — beginning tomorrow. Good luck!

REFERENCES FOR CHAPTER XI

1. Rowland, S., Report on the application of the new photography to medicine and surgery. *Br. Med. Jour.*, 1:997, 1896.

2. Stanbury, J., On the use of radioisotopes in human experimentation. *Jour. Nuc. Med.*, 11:586-591, 1970.

3. Watson, G. M., The effects of ionizing radiation on man. *Atomic Energy in Aust.*, 18:1-11, 1975.

4. National Institute for Occupational Safety and Health, Carcinogenic Properties of Ionizing and Non-ionizing Radiation. *United States* (DHEW/NIOSH Publication No.78-142), April, 1978.

5. Sternburg, J., Radiation and pregnancy. *Can. Med. Assoc. Jour.*, 109:51-57, 1973.

6. Miller, R. W., Delayed radiation effects in atomic bomb survivors. *Science*, 166:569-574, 1969.

7. Anderson, R. E., Longevity in radiated human populations, with particular reference to the atomic bomb survivors. *Amer. Jour. Med.*, 55:643-656, 1973.

8. Miller, R. W., Environmental causes of cancer in childhood. *Yr. Bk. Med. Pub. Inc.* (0065-3101/78/0025/0097), 97-119, 1978.

9. Hilberg, A. W., Use of radiation in benign diseases. *9th Annual National Conference on Radiation Control, United States* (HEW Publication), 363-368, April, 1978.

10. Morgan, K. Z., Yes is the answer to question of R.H.T. Thomas and D.D. Busick, is it really necessary to reduce patient exposure? *Amer. Ind. Hyg. Assoc. Jour.*, 37:665-668, 1976.

11. Hutchinson, G. B., Late neoplastic changes following medical irradiation. *Cancer*, 37:1102-1107, 1976.

12. Maxon, R., Thomas, S., Saenger, E., Buncher, C. and Kereiakes, J., Ionizing irradiation and the induction of clinically significant disease in the human thyroid gland. *Amer. Jour. Med.*, 63:967-978, 1977.

13. Foster, R. S., Thyroid irradiation and carcinogenesis. *Amer. Jour. Surg.*, 130:608-611, 1975.

14. Brown, J. M., Linearity vs. non-linearity of dose response for radiation carcinogenesis. *Health Physics*, 31:231-245, 1976.

15. Fry, R. J. M., and Ainsworth, E. J., Radiation injury: some aspects of the oncogenic effects. *Federation Proceedings* (Fed. Amer. Soc. for Exper. Biology), 36:1703-1707, 1977.

16. Sloan, M. H., Thyroid irradiation follow-up studies. *9th Annual National Conference on Radiation Control, United States* (HEW Publication—FDA—78-8054), 363-368, April, 1978.

17. Harley, N. H., Albert, R. E., Shore, R. E. and Pasterwack, B.S., Follow-up study of patients treated by x-ray epilation for tinea capitis. *Phys. Med. Biol.*, 21:631-642, 1976.

18. Upton, A. C., Radiobiological effects of low doses. *Radiation Research*, 71:51-74, 1977.

19. Nickson, et al, Discussion: radiation therapy. *Cancer*, 37:1108-1110, 1976.

20. White, S. C., and Frey, N. W., An estimation of somatic hazards to the United States population from dental radiography. *Oral Sur.*, 43:152-159, 1977.

21. Bond, V. P., Human radiobiology. *Crnt. Topics in Rad. Research Quart.* 9, 40-46, 1973.

22. Houston, C S., and Shokeir, M. H. K., Potential hazards of diagnostic radiation. *Jour. Can. Assoc. Radlgsts.*, 28:62-68, 1977.

23. Spar, I. L., Genetic effects of radiation. *Med. Clin. N. Amer.*, 53:965-976, 1969.

24. Morgan, K. Z., Reducing medical exposure to ionizing radiation. *Amer. Ind. Hyg. Assoc. Jour.*, 36:358-368, 1975.

25. Westmore, X-ray over use. *Scientific Australian*, July: 8-9, 1979.

26. Sternberg, J., Irradiation and radiocontamination during pregnancy. *Amer. Jour. Obstet. Gynec.*, 108:490-513, 1970.

27. Eisenbud, M., Environmental radioactivity. *Academic Press*, 1973.

28. Lundh, A., Film fogging by radiation from building materials. *Photo. Sc. Engrng.*, 18:517-523, 1974.

Appendix "A"

CHIROPRAX UNIT CALIBRATION

Unit — Chiroprax 100/100
Tube — EIMAC 316 (2.0)

1. RATIO   OF OUTPUTS WITH AND WITHOUT COLLIMATOR

80 kVp + 2 mm Al	0.826
100 kVp + 2 mm Al	0.834

2. FREE AIR OUTPUTS AT 177 cm FOR 10 x 17 FIELD

80 kVp 125 mAs	201 mR
100 kVp 50 mAs	136 mR

3. HVLs — HALF VALUE   LAYERS (Thicknesses)

80 kVp + 2 mm Al + COL.	2.5 mm Al
100 kVp + 2 mm Al + COL.	3.3 mm Al

4. RADS/ROENTGEN FACTOR 0.92 RAD/R FOR MUSCLE

5. BACKSCATTER FACTORS FOR 17 x 10 FIELD

80 kVp 2.5 mm Al HVL	1.35
100 kVp 3.3 mm Al HVL	1.4

6. ∴ PEAK SKIN DOSES WILL BE:

80 kVp 125 mAs + 2 mm Al at 177 cm for 10 x 17 field	250 mrad
100 kVp 50 mAs + 2 mm Al at 177 cm for 10 x 17 field	175 mrad

Appendix "B"

27.2.80

BACKSCATTER FACTORS

FIELD SIZE	kVp	BACKSCATTER FACTOR
43 x 25 cm, 17 x 10 inch	80	1.35
43 x 15 cm, 17 x 6 inch	80	1.33
25 x 12.5 cm, 10 x 5 inch	80	1.30
43 x 25 cm, 17 x 10 inch	100	1.40
43 x 15 cm, 17 x 6 inch	100	1.38
25 x 12.5 cm, 10 x 5 inch	100	1.35

BIBLIOGRAPHY & FURTHER READING

BOOKS

Behrens, C. F., King, E. R. and Carpenter, J. W., *Atomic Medicine*, 5th Edition. The Williams and Wilkins Co., 1969.

Christensen, E. E., Curry, T. S. and Dowdey, J. E., *An Introduction to the Physics of Diagnostic Radiology*, 2nd Edition. Lea and Febiger, 1978.

Clark, K. C., *Positioning in Radiography*, 2 Vols., 9th Edition. Published for Ilford by William Heinemann Medical Books Ltd., 1973.

Graham, B. J., and Thomas, W. N., *Physics for Radiologic Technologists*. W. B. Saunders Company, 1975.

Hendee, W. R., *Medical Radiation Physics*. Year Book Medical Publishers, 1970.

Hill, D. R., editor, *Principles of Diagnostic X-Ray Apparatus*. Philips Technical Library; the MacMillan Press Ltd., 1975.

Hiss, S. S., *Understanding Radiography*. Charles C. Thomas, 1978.

Rosenstein, M., *Organ Doses in Diagnostic Radiology*. U. S. Dept. of Health, Education and Welfare (HEW Publication—FDA—76-8030), 1976.

Schulz, R. J., *Diagnostic X-Ray Physics*. GAF Corporation, 1977.

Thompson, T. T., *A Practical Approach to Modern X-Ray Equipment*. Little, Brown and Company, 1978.

Vanderplaats, G. J., *Medical X-Ray Technique*, 3rd Edition. Philips Technical Library; Centrex Publishing, 1969.

JOURNALS

Barnes, G. T., The dependence of radiographic mottle on beam quality. *American Jour. Roentgenology*, 127:819-24, 1976.

Becker, J., Adjustable compensating filters for pediatric 72-inch spine radiography. *Radiologic Technology*, 51:11-15, 1979.

Buchanan, R. A., Finkelstein, S. E. and Wickersheim, K. A., X-ray exposure reduction using rare earth oxysulfide intensifying screens. *Radiology*, 105:185-90, 1972.

Castle, J. W., Sensitivity of radiographic screens to scattered radiation and its relationship to image contrast. *Radiology*, 122:805-09, 1977.

Jackson, W., Filtration in diagnostic radiology. *Radiography*, 42:255-60, 1976.

Lundh, A., Film fogging by radiation from building materials. *Photographic Science and Engineering*, 18:517-23, 1974.

Roberts, F. F., Kishore, P. R. and Cunningham, M E., Routine oblique radiography of the pediatric lumbar spine: is it necessary? *American Journal Roentgenology*, 131:297-98, 1978.

Rossi, R. P., Hendee, W. R. and Ahrens, C. R., An evaluation of rare earth screen/film combinations. *Radiology*, 121:465-71, 1976.

Sackett, M. H., Caution: speed ahead—rare earth imaging systems. *Radiologic Technology*, 48:537-43, 1977.

Stevels, A. L., New Phosphors for x-ray screens. *Medicamundi*, 20: 12-22, 1975.

Venema, H. W., X-ray absorption, speed and luminescent efficiency of rare earth and other intensifying screens. *Radiology*, 130:765-71, 1979.

Villagran, J. E., Hobbs, B. B. and Taylor, K. W., Reduction of patient exposure by use of heavy elements as radiation filters in diagnostic radiology. *Radiology,* 127:249-54, 1978.

Wagner, R. F., and Weaver, K. E., Prospects for x-ray exposure reduction using rare earth intensifying screens, *Radiology,* 118:183-88, 1976.

Wilson, B. C., and Sage M. R., Radiation doses in computerized tomography. *Medical Journal Australia,* 2:30-32, 1979.

OTHER MATERIAL

AGFA-Gevaert Mortsel, Series of "training department roentgen" monographs, 1975, 1976.

Dupont Photo Products Department (Australia), Resident lecture series supplement.

Eastman Kodak Company, The fundamentals of radiography, 11th Edition. 1968.

Siemans Aktiengesellschaft, Medical engineering formulae facts, 1979.

INDEX